T3-BNX-343

DATE DUE

How Many Roads...?

Queen's-CMA Conference on Regionalization & Decentralization in Health Care

Edited by
John L. Dorland
S. Mathwin Davis

Canadian Cataloguing in Publication Data

Main entry under title:

How many roads--? : regionalization and decentralization in health care

Proceedings of a conference held in Kingston, Ont. in June, 1995.
ISBN 0-88911-713-6

1. Regional medical program – Canada – Congresses.
2. Medical policy – Canada – Congresses. I. Dorland, John, 1946-
II. Davis, Sturton Mathwin, 1919-   . III. Queen's University
(Kingston, Ont.). School of Policy Studies.

RA449.H68 1996   362.1'0971   C96-930076-X

to my daughters
Katherine and Alexandra
from whom I learn
more each day

JLD

to my grand-daughters
Catherine and Anne Munier

SMD

Contents

PRACTICAL CONSIDERATIONS

APPENDIX

Tables and Figures

Tables

Figures

Acknowledgements

When, as in this instance, the School of Policy Studies at Queen's has arranged previous health policy conferences — it is fairly easy for one or two individuals to say "Let's have another one." Like a stone thrown into a pool, however, this initial splash must lead to a series of expanding ripples before the conference becomes a reality. It is essential therefore to express appreciation to all those whose varied endeavours over several months have made possible what *has* been described as a successful conference.

First then — and perhaps most importantly — we must thank all those who felt it was worthwhile to attend and were prepared to make the outlay of time and expense to do so. Without their involvement the conference would have been an empty shell.

In the overall, and somewhat lengthy, effort of planning it is important to acknowledge the direct cooperation of the Canadian Medical Association as well as the ongoing involvement of Queen's Health Policy, the Kingston, Frontenac and Lennox & Addington — Queen's Teaching Health Unit, and the Canadian Health Economics Research Association. A Working Group from these activities laboured for over 12 months with a wealth of conceptual and administrative detail. As well as appreciating their efforts, we must also take note of the high quality of the speakers they were able to attract, as well as the informative papers that were presented.

While the foregoing takes note of the intellectual aspects of the conference, due recognition must also be given to those who provided the essential financial support — without which the conference could not have been mounted. Thus, we are happy to recognize the very substantial financial contributions from the Canadian Medical Association, Health Canada and the Ministry of Health — Ontario, as well as from the Kingston, Frontenac and Lennox & Addington Health Unit. Equally appreciated were sponsorships of speakers from Glaxo-Wellcome, Kingston General Hospital, and MDS Health Groups Inc.

No less important to the success of any conference are the efforts of those who labour, generally unseen, in the myriad of administrative chores that demand careful attention. Here, we particularly appreciate the organizational skills of Shelley Pilon of SeaShell Consulting, and the unobtrusive but significant contributions from staff members of the School of Policy Studies — Lynn Freeman, Marilyn Redmond, and especially Jane Hodgins. The design skills of Mark Howes and Valerie Jarus of the Publication Unit of the School were also valuable.

Most especially, we would like to express the warmest appreciation for the editorial and production efforts of Marilyn Banting. Her skilled assistance was essential in producing this comprehensive report.

Thus, any errors must quite clearly be assigned to the co-editors.

John L. Dorland
S. Mathwin Davis
1996

Organizing Committee

Owen Adams
Canadian Medical Association

S. Mathwin Davis
School of Policy Studies
Queen's University

John L. Dorland
Queen's Health Policy
Queen's University

Fleur-Ange Lefebvre
Canadian Medical Association

David Mowat
Kingston, Frontenac, Lennox &
Addington Health Unit

Shelley Pilon
SeaShell Consulting

Art Stewart
School of Policy Studies
Queen's University

Bill Swan
Queen's Health Policy
CHERA/ACRES

Bill Tholl
Canadian Medical Association

Opening Remarks

Duncan G. Sinclair

There are few topics more contemporary or important in Canada in this last half-decade of the twentieth century. In nine of the ten provinces of this country, regional health authorities are operating in one form or another, some for just a few months but others, notably in the province of Quebec, for many years. These authorities represent attempts by central governments to come to grips with the reality that all of the provinces have run out of money and that in health care, as in many other sectors of publicly-funded endeavours, very difficult choices have become necessary. Such choices are extremely difficult to make centrally, especially in those provinces with substantial populations or in those with substantial geographic and demographic diversity — such as those where travel is very difficult, especially in winter.

Regionalization and decentralization are organizational devices to shift governance — by definition, to govern is to make choices — from the centre to the regional populations which are most directly affected by the outcome of setting priorities and making choices accordingly. The theory is very sound. Those primarily affected by decisions should be most closely involved in making them. In practice, however, there are some unanswered questions such as:

- How are the members of regional health authorities held accountable by the populations they are said to represent?
- What are the tolerable limits of variation in the outcomes of decisions on the availability of health-care services, region by region?

- What are the *real* limits available for decisionmaking by regional health authorities within the guidelines and management supervision imposed by central government?

- Where do we find people in our regions with the experience in governance, for membership on the boards of public sector institutions and agencies, and to take responsibility as directors/governors on regional health authorities?

There are many such questions. Many of them will be dealt with over the life of the conference. This is the first and most important step in finding the answers we need urgently as we approach the new dawn of fiscal realities in this last five years of the 1990s.

Léo Paul Landry

The Queen's-CMA Conference on Regionalization and Decentralization in Health Care comes at a time of unprecedented changes in the Canadian health system — changes in both its structure and organization. Regionalization initiatives across Canada (and, indeed, internationally) are a major vehicle for these changes.

Change, especially in an area as important as health care, is always difficult. As Will Rogers once said: "Everybody likes progress; it's the changes they don't like!" But if we are to make progress in meeting the evolving health needs of Canadians, change we must. I say *we* because, if the changes are to be meaningful and stand the test of time, it must be a shared effort channelled in pursuit of shared objectives.

The Canadian Medical Association is committed to doing its part to help manage change in health care, today and into the future. Our commitment to facilitating and, yes, leading change is also reflected in our research efforts in the whole arena of regionalization. In the spring of 1991 the board of directors of the CMA authorized a major research undertaking in regionalization. This research endeavour involved in-depth interviews with key informants having "hands-on" experience in regionalization, both here in Canada and abroad — 85 experts in all. This work resulted in the release of the CMA report entitled *The Language of Health System Reform* in the fall of 1993.

We are currently in the process of updating this report, and we are completing a survey of the effects of regionalization on physicians' practices in facilities and community practice; this survey was administered to key informants in regional health authorities, ministries of health, and other organizations.

In May 1995, the CMA board approved a "Policy Position Paper on Regionalization of Health Services in Canada." This paper builds on the research findings contained in *The Language of Health System Reform* and goes on to develop policy principles that are intended to guide regionalization strategies and to help shape the assignment of authority, accountability, and resource control over health-service delivery in Canada from the perspective of the medical profession. The guiding policy principles identified in the document address the topics of: clear statements of objectives in the development and implementation of regionalization strategies; accountability and authority; needs-based planning; informed choice; participatory democracy; clinical autonomy; evaluation; standards for reasonable access; and balancing access and affordability.

When we began our work on regionalization in early 1991, I think it is fair to say that only Quebec had announced its plans for a significant expansion of regionalization in the *Reform Centred on the Citizen*. Since that time, virtually every provincial jurisdiction has put in place some form of regionalized structure. These initiatives have proceeded at an almost dizzying pace.

While a wealth of documentation has been generated, including enabling legislation, guides and manuals on how to implement regionalization, and cross-country scans, there is nothing like learning first-hand from those who have been directly involved with introducing, implementing, managing, and assessing regionalization initiatives — hence, a conference such as this that brings together government representatives, academics, administrators, health-care providers, and consumers is very important.

It is our hope that the Queen's-CMA Conference on Regionalization and Decentralization in Health Care will add to our collective knowledge-base on regionalization efforts. I look forward to meeting other involved and committed individuals, and to working with them to make a good system better. The Canadian public expects, and deserves, nothing less.

INTRODUCTION

1

Regionalization as Health-Care Reform

John L. Dorland and S. Mathwin Davis

The Canadian health-care system is often lauded as being the best in the world and, equally as often, declared to be in mortal crisis. Both statements are perhaps hyperbolical, but like all hyperboles, contain a central core of truth. We do have an excellent health-care system, which compares favourably with any in the world on many measures. However, it is not a static system, nor does it exist in a static social and economic environment. We cannot relax our attention and expect the system to retain its excellence. Continued excellence requires continual examination, evaluation, and frequent change. This conference, co-sponsored by Queen's University and the Canadian Medical Association, has been held in the spirit of continual examination, evaluation and improvement in the Canadian health-care system.

As many of the speakers reminded us, this need for evaluation and change is neither recent nor particular to Canada's health-care system. Most of the world's health-care systems have been under serious scrutiny over the past decade; many have been undergoing various degrees of reform and re-reform, even before any major changes were contemplated in Canada. However, the tides of change have now definitely reached Canadian shores. Every province is now either in the midst of, or about to embark upon major health-care reforms.

Although individual countries around the world have taken widely different approaches to organizing (or not) their health-care systems, there has been one near-universal element of reform, which is (to use the term broadly at this point) the regionalization of health-care systems. Because of its universal importance, we chose this as the theme of our conference. Our approach to this theme was to build upon the accumulating experience of many countries and provinces with regionalization reforms and to emphasize the expected outcomes and evaluation of the reforms. To that end, our panel of speakers included academics, politicians, government officials and senior managers from several countries and from many Canadian provinces, all of whom brought their experience and expertise with health-care regionalization to the conference. In keeping with its practical orientation, we also identified six sub-topics of crucial importance to the implementation of regionalization, and conducted small-group workshops on these topics, led by expert faculty.

In addition to its appeal as a worldwide reform phenomenon, health-care regionalization has a special interest in the Canadian context, for two reasons. The first is that Canada already has a regionalized health-care system, built around the federal-provincial government structure. This raises interesting questions such as: How is this "new" regionalization different from the original regionalization? Is this a search for an optimum geographic size or population base for efficient health-care systems? The second reason is somewhat more abstract, and is related to the origins of the Canadian system. Historically, the Canadian health-care "system" was largely a matter of local public initiative, based upon municipal hospitals and other charitable and religious institutions. As medical care became more complex, effective, expensive and socially important, the responsibility for the system was centralized (at the provincial level) in a large public bureaucracy. One of the rationales for creating this centralized publicly administered health-care system was the recognition that in making decisions about health-care issues, people had a considerable knowledge deficit, and needed a strong central authority to make decisions in the public interest. Now, after 25 years, regionalization reforms are creating smaller decisionmaking units, with (in theory) much more public involvement. Thus, the reforms have the appealing apparent objective, at least on the surface, of returning the system to local interests. This also raises interesting questions, such as: Does this reflect the attainment of a higher level of maturity in the system and in the population? What is the nature and success of the increased public involvement?

The conference papers have been grouped into two major sections. The *Context of Reform* section contains four papers which provide the historical, political, legal, and conceptual background for the discussion of regionalization reforms. The second major section, *Practical Considerations*, includes papers that examine specific regionalization reforms which have been implemented in Canada and several other countries.

So much for background. How then did the conference unfold? In the first plenary session, David Peterson, from his vantage point as a recent former premier of Ontario, raised several interesting questions and offered some helpful warnings. He observed that the "population" which the health-care system now serves is not the same population as a decade ago. The demographic changes are well-known, but more importantly, attitudes and expectations have also changed dramatically, and perhaps even core values. In fact, one must ask if medicare itself is still included in these core values? Mr. Peterson stated that the time seemed right for fundamental reforms which changed the underlying incentives in the system, but warned against apparent reforms that merely shifted political flak from one level to another. With regard to the implementation of reforms, he challenged policymakers not to analyze forever, but to just do it.

In another paper which provided context for the conference, Marie Fortier reminded us that the federal government is still a major player in the health-care system, and reviewed the various instruments of influence which define the relationship between the federal and provincial governments in the health-care field.

Jonathan Lomas' paper provided us with the language of regionalization with a precision and insight that permitted distinction and comparison among the various models. One of his findings, both counter-intuitive and illuminating, was that regionalization reforms, which always affect the transfer of some degree of power from a central authority to a smaller geograhical/population base, also generally involve an element of centralization, in that powers formerly at the local level may be concentrated upwards to a new regional level. Mr. Lomas' paper also provided an early look at the characteristics and attitudes of the people who are exercising these new regional powers in Canada.

In the final paper in this section, Richard Fraser addressed the legal, philosophical and practical aspects of accountability and liability in regionalized health-care systems. He foresees, perhaps unfortunately, increased litigation as a result of regionalization, extending beyond the issue of medical malpractice (to which the courts have always been receptive) into areas such as inadequate system design, negligent provision of care, and inappropriate resource allocation. Mr. Fraser also noted the great effect that system structure can have on the relationships within the system and the way accountability is discharged.

Papers by Alan Maynard, Raisa Deber, and Malcolm Anderson described the international experience with regionalization reforms, with emphasis on the United Kingdom, Northern Europe, and New Zealand respectively. Reforms in these countries have centred around the establishment and management of regional "markets" for health-care services. These managed markets vary widely in size, regulatory structure and operation, but derive from a common underlying conviction that the market mechanism will automatically lead to greater efficiency, equity, and cost containment.

The reforms have usually been implemented with much political enthusiasm, and have undoubtedly generated a great deal of "change." Whether these changes represent progress is not so clear. In general, objectives (beyond cost containment) have not been clearly specified, and accordingly evaluation results have been thin or contentious.

The more recent Canadian experience was described in papers by Russell King, Paul Lamarche, Alan Warren, and John Malcom, addressing primarily New Brunswick, Quebec, Ontario, and Saskatchewan. The variety of approaches even within Canada is striking. Ontario, with the largest population, has not moved from a relatively weak regional planning model implemented in the 1970s, while several smaller provinces, including Saskatchewan, have enthusiastically transferred population-based budgets and allocation powers to smaller regional authorities. Like the international models, these reforms appear to be driven primarily on ideological conviction. Evidence of effectiveness in achieving specific objectives is still non-existent, although it is early days for most of the Canadian reforms.

The Roundtable included presentations from payers, providers, and the community. These raised concerns regarding the need to emphasize the health of the population as a whole, with a requirement for training to respond to the labour market adjustments involved. It was held to be important that providers — with their relevant experience — should not be excluded from the decisionmaking process.

However, noting the necessity for effective communication, the selection of representative regional boards was seen as critical. It was important that such boards should concentrate on overall supervision and representation of community interests, with micro-management being left to professionals.

Looking back over the conference, what should we conclude? The major conclusion must be that, despite worldwide experimentation with regional models, and with years of accumulated experience in some jurisdictions, major conclusions are still not possible. For many reforms, clear expectations and objectives have never been specified, and evaluation results are extremely thin. However, it is abundantly clear that this type of reform has captured the imagination of policymakers everywhere, and has stimulated a great deal of enthusiastic, energetic change in the system. As a reform movement, regionalization in its many variations has conformed to David Peterson's challenge that when change is necessary, one should not analyze forever, but "just do it." Having "just done it," however, it is now imperative that we observe and analyze the consequences of what we have done, to appraise the results against reasonable objectives, and to ensure that we progress, not merely change. It is this task that now falls to all of us.

CONTEXT OF REFORM

2

Reflections on Medicare as a National Institution

David Peterson

Let me say at the outset that while I have no professional expertise in your field, I would like to share some reflections of one who has gone through the health-care war, who has wrestled with some of the problems and, in many respects, have found the "solutions" to be wanting. Undoubtedly, this is probably the most complex policy area that any government deals with — and more so now than in the past. We need to recall that, in the late 1980s we were sitting in an age of unparalleled plenty in this province, in the midst of a widespread industrial boom, but that, even then, a wide range of problems were building. It has often been said that if one seeks to change things you probably have to wait for a crisis — so that people are prepared to accept change. I suspect, indeed, that we are now in that crisis situation.

There are, it seems to me, a number of contemporary problems or constraints that, together, are enhancing our difficulties. Let me enunciate some of these:

Demography. The aging population will bring great pressures, not just on health care but in the entire welfare area, the income security area and others.

Diseases. With our increased ability to diagnose, as well as the onset of new social maladies, we are facing the spectre of new and expensive diseases.

Technology. With the benefit of research and new concepts, there is a burgeoning of new and expensive technologies whose distribution represents demanding ethical concerns.

Consumers. Undoubtedly, with greater knowledge and a concern for human rights, health-care consumers are becoming more aggressive with demands for a greater choice.

Unfortunately, in my experience, there was a health ministry lacking a plan of any substance, generally driven by providers more than consumers and with a tendency to respond to political challenges and demands. Undoubtedly the range of providers were good people and well motivated but everybody wanted nothing less than "the best." And, from a political viewpoint it was easier to accept a measure of duplication rather than attempting to mediate between competing institutions.

Nevertheless, I believe there is the more fundamental question of whether or not medicare *is* a core value of society. This has clearly been a fundamental belief — or perhaps a mythology — and it is not clear that we can continue to accept its tenets. We cannot avoid considering the overall cost of our health care — the second most expensive system in the world and one that has been growing dramatically and excessively. With no checks on the consumer, who has unlimited access to the system, there are obvious limits to our capacity to fund this on an ongoing basis, but no way to constrain the system.

Notwithstanding the foregoing excesses it has to be recognized that people generally are now more demanding, more sensitive to the desire of value for money and very ready to change allegiances — politically or institutionally — when it appears advantageous. In such a "retail revolution" there has been a growing need to remove "margins" from a wide range of activities with providers needing to be more creative, more efficient and prepared to work harder and more cheaply in order to survive. In the health sector an example is provided by the laboratories in hospitals which appear to be far more expensive to run than those operating in the private sector. It would seem that privatization is an obvious solution in this instance.

This leads me to a broader consideration of the health-care system. Here, as in society generally, there is a greater overall concern for effectiveness, with a need to concentrate on successful outputs rather than simply considering inputs. Fortunately we are becoming more sophisticated in these matters — but a more informed public will demand results. However, it has long been my view that the incentives in the health-care system are totally perverse and antithetical to human behaviour. Indeed, it would appear that all the incentives are to consume than the reverse. Perhaps the drug benefit plan is a good example of this, where a prescription with a pharmacist's fee is sometimes suggested as a preferred alternative to an over-the-counter drug. There is no *incentive* here to take the low-cost option. Similarly, with the somewhat cherished fee-for-service payment of physicians which may well lead to an excessive number of consultations. In my view, we are going to see more capitation and will have to face the conflicts about who will be assigned what portion of the population. Similarly with the changing roles for hospitals as there is a move from institutionalized to non-institutionalized care.

The situation is somewhat analogous to that of the banks where — with the extensive use of cash-machines — there is less need for the existing infrastructure. In the case of hospitals, there has, so far, been a tendency to meet the problem by a general reduction of hospital *beds*. The hospitals themselves, however, remain with boards, administrative structures, and the like. It seems to me that we must broaden into complete health-care areas with local responsibility for total health-care outcomes.

Let me return though to the basic question of incentives. People are infinitely adaptable and, given changing circumstances will undoubtedly — as provider or consumer — seek to maximize their own positions and benefits. Thus, those seeking to make decisions must seriously consider the development of incentives that can harness the reality of human nature and concentrate on outputs and results, rather than a gloomy realization of growing inputs.

As a concluding theme, I would like to give consideration to the topic of governance. This has been the subject of much discussion with varied models, but I am left with the question: Are the models more efficient or are they simply for shifting political flack? Like most ministries, Health does not like undue public grief. And yet, when any entity comes forward — well intentioned undoubtedly and with first-rate motivation — they are concerned solely with their own benefit and care little for other activities in this province. These broader issues are not their concern. Thus, when we contemplate regionalization we must take care not to devolve so much responsibility that there can be no balancing between regions. Within a given region, however, it may well be desirable to let the local authority make the difficult apportionments among the various elements of health care. Nevertheless, in any devolution system a particular effort must be made to keep the various bureaucratic layers to an absolute minimum. This, of course, is not to say that the division into appropriate regions is going to be simple or straightforward.

It has often been said that the government which is closest to the people probably works best in making hard choices and bearing the responsibility for them. But we must not conclude that this will relieve the Ministry of Health of all its responsibilities — they are the ones that ultimately must pay and be accountable.

In conclusion therefore, I repeat my conviction that you can introduce change at two times — when all is quiet and successful *or* when there is a sense of crisis. I believe that, right now, we are close enough to a sense of crisis that the time is ripe for a change in the health-care system. In particular, the political mood is ripe for change. Five years ago governments could succeed, in an age of 'plenty,' by promising to spend more to solve every social problem. Today there are far *more* social problems, but the concern has shifted to cutting deficits, reducing taxes, and seeking efficiency in government. Indeed, the issue of the deficit and of government finances generally is becoming a serious issue for average citizens. Generally, they are prepared to take the cuts and to accept changes in the system. Thus, I encourage you to go forward with courage, to make decisions and to see that these decisions are implemented. Do not look for perfect solutions — these will never appear — but *do* seize the opportunity, go ahead, make the necessary decisions and take responsibility for them. Probably there will not be another time that is so ripe for change as the present and that presents an invaluable opportunity to make a substantial difference.

I believe that medicare *is* a core value, that it represents the gentleness and the sharing and the respect for diversity that this country embraces. But we have to understand that core values *do* change and we have to try and ensure that medicare, perhaps in a somewhat different form, will remain and — with particular efforts — even be enhanced.

3

The Evolving Federal Role
in Health Care

Marie Fortier

This paper is about some of the opportunities and challenges that face
Canada's health-care system and the work that is being done to address
these issues.

I will outline very briefly what some of these challenges and potential
new directions are, the federal role in addressing them, some of the levers
it has at its disposal to do so, and the steps that the National Forum on
Health is taking to assist in this area.

The topic of the federal role in health is of particular interest to the
Forum right now, and our working group on Striking a Balance is examining it as part of its work on how best to use resources to improve health and
health care.

THE FEDERAL ROLE IN HEALTH

For many Canadians, federal and provincial responsibility for health is
blurred; polls in fact show that there is little general awareness of the divisions of responsibility between governments. It may be useful here to give

an overview of the federal role, given its particular complexities. It is fair to say that, while the provinces are the primary deliverers of health care, the federal government has a strong presence in the field of health, and this presence is enshrined both in the constitution and in the practices and precedents that have been established — especially in the last 40 years.

In fact, the high standard of health care we enjoy in this country is the result of the strong partnerships that have evolved between the federal and provincial/territorial governments since the 1950s and 1960s when our current system was established. The federal role in health derives first from the constitution.

THE CONSTITUTION AND SOURCES OF FEDERAL POWER IN HEALTH

The constitution is less precise about the division of powers in health than most people realize. This reflects a distinction between health and health care. The provinces are responsible for delivering health care to the majority of Canadians, but the federal government has a number of constitutional powers in areas that affect health. And, even in the relatively narrow field of health care proper, the exercise of spending power in support of the *Canada Health Act* is not without foundation.

The three main areas of constitutional power are criminal law, spending power, and peace, order and good government.

Criminal law is one of the most straightforward of the powers. It is the basis, for example, of the *Narcotics Control Act* and the *Food and Drug Act,* both of which have a large impact on health.

The second is *spending power.* The constitution gives the federal government the power to levy taxes and appropriate funds. This could have been narrowly interpreted to restrict spending power only to areas within federal jurisdiction, but that would have condemned the poorer provinces to either higher levels of taxation or lower levels of services. Early legislation, such as the *Old Age Pension Act*, provided precedents for a broader interpretation.

In fact, the federal government makes major transfers to the provinces and territories to help them to meet their health care and other mandates.

Third, the *peace, order and good government* clause of the constitution gives the federal government authority to address areas of national concern and emergencies or crises. The "national concern" doctrine gives the federal government the authority to maintain and improve countrywide standards, not just in health, but also in other areas that have an impact on health, such as air and water quality.

THE CURRENT FEDERAL ROLE

The current federal role, which derives from these constitutional powers and from historical and practical considerations, falls into four broad areas of responsibility: the first, and most direct, is the delivery of health-care services to specific groups of people. These include primary care to First Nations people on reserves, and some services to the RCMP, Correctional Services, the Armed Forces, and veterans.

The second area falls under the broad category of protecting the health of Canadians. The minister of health serves as a health advisor to Canadians on issues of importance and concern to them. In this role, the minister — directly or in cooperation with other federal agencies and provincial governments — sets standards and guidelines and ensures that Canadians have accurate and timely health information on which to base individual choices and decisions. For example, Health Canada regulates the safety and efficacy of drugs and medical devices; the Department of Fisheries and Oceans monitors the safety of the fish and seafood we buy; and Environment Canada watches over our land, air, and water quality.

The third area of federal responsibility is support of the health-care system. This includes instruments such as the *Canada Health Act,* federal-provincial transfers, and research funding. Transfer payments can take many forms. For example, they can be transfers to provinces, individuals, or organizations; they can be equalized or non-equalized. They can be in the form of cash and/or tax points (some argue that tax points are one-time transfers), block-funding and cost-sharing, and subsidies. They can be conditional or non-conditional. This, of course, is an extremely large and important area and it is one I will come back to later.

The fourth area of federal responsibility in health is to promote strategies to improve the health of the population. These strategies — in areas such as health promotion, illness prevention, and education — represent a comprehensive set of activities to mobilize others to educate, inform, and encourage individuals to take an active part in enhancing their own health and well-being. This responsibility, too, cuts across several departments, including Human Resources Development.

To carry out these broad responsibilities the federal government has a number of tools or levers at its disposal. They include:

- various tax measures that impact on the health system such as the medical expense credit and the exemption for employer-sponsored health benefit plans;
- its role as a leader and national coordinator, and partner with the provinces in fostering national approaches and exercising moral suasion;
- legislation in the form of the *Canada Health Act* and regulatory mandates in areas such as food and drugs, medical devices, hazardous products, and the environment;
- significant work in research and evaluation represents another important lever. The federal government leads the way in support of health research primarily through the Medical Research Council and the National Health Research and Development Program. In related areas, the federal government supports the Social Sciences and Humanities Research Council, the Natural Sciences and Engineering Research Council and the National Research Council.
- international responsibilities: responding to the "internationalization" of disease, technology, and standards; and
- direct spending on specific programs and initiatives such as Brighter Futures, Family Violence, Aids.

WHY EXAMINE THE FEDERAL ROLE NOW?

The federal role and activities in health and health care are important, pervasive, and have a long history, which begs the question: Why then examine the federal role at all?

Clearly, these are extraordinary times for health and health care. Canadians are concerned about their health, the health-care system and the *Canada Health Act.* In every province, the health-care system is undergoing major reform. Budgets are facing immense reductions and the health-care system is being reconfigured in many ways. Further, the paradigm is shifting from medical care to health, from curative to disease prevention and rehabilitation. Consumers are expected to assume greater responsibility for their own health care at a time when the numbers, mix, and roles of health-care providers are changing.

There is a fear that the federal government will lose control — that the health system Canadians have come to cherish will be eroded. And, it is clear that some of this fear was sparked by the most recent federal budget and the changes that will be brought to the system of transfers to provinces through the Canada Health and Social Transfer.

In order to put this in context, I need to go back a bit. Federal involvement in the financing of health and postsecondary education (PSE) dates back to the immediate postwar period when grants were established for the education of returning veterans and for construction of hospitals and assistance for medical schools. In the 1950s, these arrangements were replaced by more generalized grants to educational institutions and by cost-sharing of provincial hospital insurance programs.

The trend toward cost-sharing continued into the 1960s with the shift to federal sharing of institutional PSE costs in 1967 and the introduction of medicare in 1968. The introduction of Established Programs Financing in 1977 resulted in the replacement of health and the PSE cost-sharing by a formula yielding an initially equal per capita block-fund transfer to all provinces. The EPF arrangements provided federal financial assistance to the provinces and territories in respect of insured health services, extended health-care services (EHCS) and postsecondary education. Although the transfer was notionally earmarked for health (67.9 percent of transfer) and postsecondary education (32.1 percent) provinces were not bound to spend the money in this manner; payments flowed into the provinces' Consolidated Revenue Funds.

The introduction of the original EPF block-funding formula meant that transfers to the provinces would take the form of cash payments (basic cash) and tax points, the latter involving a reduction of federal tax with a concomitant and equal increase in provincial tax. Increases in funding were provided for in the 1977 formula based on GNP and population growth. The original formula was locked in for five years (1977 to 1982). There have been a number of funding formula changes and freezes to EPF since that time. First, a significant change to the funding formula in 1982 meant that cash payments (basic cash) would eventually be squeezed out as the value of the tax point transfer increases. In other words, financial assistance from the federal government in terms of hard cash would eventually be eliminated. Successive budgets since 1986 have reduced the rate of growth of the total transfer and eventually frozen the per capita amount.

The 1995 federal budget announced that the Canada Health and Social Transfer (CHST) would be a new federal-provincial transfer program that would combine social and health transfers to the provinces. This new CHST would be a block fund, leaving the provinces free to determine how the resources should be allocated. Total funding to provinces under CHST would be reduced by $2.5 billion in 1996-97 compared to projected transfer entitlements under the existing set of programs; and by $4.5 billion in 1997-98.

These developments will have an impact on provincial finances, and, in the longer term could affect the federal government's ability to maintain the principles of the *Canada Health Act*. The concern that is being voiced in terms of the Act is that if the cash component of the CHST is allowed to dwindle or disappear, the federal government will lose its leverage in the health field.

Bill C-76 was passed in the House of Commons on 6 June 1995. I just want to make a few points of clarification about its effects. First, Bill C-76 is not the final definition of what the Canada Health and Social Transfer will be. It is interim legislation which will allow for a process to unfold and for negotiations with the provinces to proceed in the fall.

Second, the question of the cash reaching zero is not an immediate problem. Assuming the current situation, cash would not run out for at least ten years. In the meantime the federal government will consult with provinces and territories in developing a permanent method of allocation. This allocation formula will govern the payments after the first year. The size and allocation of the cash component will be addressed during these discussions.

Third, CHST maintains the ties to the *Canada Health Act*. The principles of the Act will continue to apply. The work of the Forum in this regard is, therefore, still timely and relevant.

SO WHAT CAN THE FORUM CONTRIBUTE TO THIS ISSUE?

The Forum's job is to engage and guide the debate surrounding our future health and health-care system, and to help find ways to reshape the system so that it remains universal, accessible, comprehensive, portable, and publicly funded. As part of this job, the Forum is examining the current federal role in the two areas that fall under its mandate — improving the health of the population and supporting the health-care system.

Canadians have a profound and fundamental belief in their health-care system. They know it is one of the finest in the world. Several polls and other research projects give us some insight into this aspect. We know that Canadians feel strongly about medicare. A 1994 Ekos Research Associates Inc. poll revealed that Canadians rank health third in a list of 22 values that they believe the federal government should uphold (behind maintaining freedom and a clean environment). Medicare is the most popular public program in Canada and 79 percent of the population count on the federal government to save it.

Many Canadians see it as a distinguishing feature of who they are in a global village whose boundaries are increasingly blurred. They need to be reassured that there are cost-effective ways to maintain the integrity of the system while reducing costs. Only by putting all the cards on the table — by opening discussion to include all possible aspects of health, medicare, and the role of the federal government — can we have the transparency and fruitful discussion we need to achieve the best possible long-term results.

Because federal-provincial transfers are such a defining feature of the federal role in health, we will focus considerable attention on this aspect. We will review the historical perspective of transfers, recent restraint measures, and implications for the federal role. We will also review their effectiveness in enforcing national standards, will draw out possible scenarios for the future, and assess options — including the use of other levers — to enforce national principles. Criteria for evaluating the effectiveness of various levers might include how they work in controlling the growth of health costs (public and private); maintaining or improving the quality and effectiveness of health services; and preventing undue fragmentation of the health system; their cost and ease of administration, their legal standing, and the impact of their use on federal-provincial relations.

In addition to studying our own system, we will also examine levers in other countries to see if Canada can learn from their experience. Particular attention will be devoted to the social and political context in which these levers are exercised.

As I mentioned at the beginning, this task of assessing federal levers falls to the Striking a Balance working group. The group will also undertake other projects in its investigation of the best use of resources to improve health, within and outside the health system. These other projects include: a study of international and interprovincial data on health and social expenditures, service utilization, health status, and other indicators to find meaningful differences that could lead to new ideas; a review of the issues of public/private financing of health services and the development of a framework that might be used to determine classes of services which should be covered and what their financing sources should be; and an examination of barriers and strategies for change and various decentralization and regionalization models.

CONCLUSION

Other working groups are focusing their projects on three complementary issues:

- how to improve the foundations on which decisions about health are made;
- how to create for Canadians the conditions which are most conducive to health; and

- identifying the values held by Canadians with respect to health and deciding how they can be articulated.

The Forum has a great deal of work ahead. It is putting forward some big questions and will be asking all Canadians — experts and the general public — to contribute to the answers. Dialogue is key to the Forum's work. We are developing a process that will encourage input from a large number of sources and, at the same time, expand knowledge and understanding of the issues.

As the country looks ahead to a revitalized health-care system and new ways of ensuring the health of its population, it is imperative that we also assess the role of the federal government in meeting these objectives. Only by periodically reviewing the strong, solid partnerships among levels of government and other stakeholders can we ensure that Canadians continue to enjoy one of the highest standards of health in the world.

4

Devolved Authorities in Canada: The New Site of Health-Care System Conflict?

Jonathan Lomas

CANADA'S REGIONALIZATION POLICY IN INTERNATIONAL PERSPECTIVE

A review of the numerous health reform task force and royal commission reports that flowed from the provinces in the late 1980s and early 1990s reveals a large number of common themes. Indeed, the commonality of these themes is international, not just domestic. Health-care systems around the world are grappling with the same challenges:

- cost containment
- improved health outcomes
- increased flexibility and responsiveness in delivery of care
- better integration and coordination of services.

In many Western European countries and New Zealand, governments have put their faith in the purchaser-provider split as the policy vehicle most likely to meet the challenge. The providers in these countries are being asked to compete with each other, largely on the basis of price and quality, in order to encourage government or government-designated payers to choose to contract with them for the delivery of services. The experiences of those countries that have chosen devolved authorities as the purchasers are described later in Chapter 6. In the United States and a few of the Western European countries such as Germany, the chosen policy vehicle has been managed competition. Here, the intent is to encourage the payers to compete with each other on the basis of the price, quality and scope of the complete "insurance package" they offer to "consumers" (either individuals or employers). Both these policy avenues rely on competition and some regulated concept of "market" to achieve their aims, but in one case it is competition between providers and in the other it is competition between payers.

In Canada we have, so far, chosen to shun this new Jerusalem of competition and markets, perhaps influenced more than other countries by our proximity to the United States — home of the prolonged failure of market-driven health policy panaceas. Instead, Canada has chosen to retain our historic reliance on "command and control" regulation coupled, however, in all but a couple of provinces, with a reconfigured and more local site from which at least some of the commands and controls emanate. It is not that the development of these new devolved authorities is incompatible with a purchaser-provider split approach (although their monopoly status does make them incompatible with managed competition), but rather that provinces have not chosen (yet) to exploit this potential addition to the reform. Instead, the aforementioned task forces and commissions seem to have seen devolved bodies as ways of increasing community involvement and public participation and, therefore, as instrumental vehicles leading to improvements in cost containment, health outcomes, flexibility and responsiveness, and integration and coordination.

DEVOLVED AUTHORITY AS AN ONGOING NEGOTIATION

This policy of "devolved command and control" has created more than 100 new regional or local bodies in Canada, with powers and scopes of authority that vary from limited power over hospitals (New Brunswick) to extensive resource allocation and other powers over a combined budget for community services, welfare, housing, corrections, and almost all health care (Prince Edward Island).[1] In addition to choosing what functions (if any) to delegate (e.g., planning, management, resource allocation, delivery, and so on), each province has had to choose where to situate its formal design on at least three other dimensions:

Where?

At what geographic level is "the system" defined: the provincial, the regional or the local?

What?

The breadth of service choice and allocation decisions over which authority will exist, that is, the scope of the defined system: limited health-care programs, all health-care programs, health care and social services, or "health-related investments" (e.g., housing).

Who?

Whose values and what information will be used to inform program choices and resource allocations: provincial politicians/bureaucrats and (potentially) major stakeholder interests, administrators and planners, or community appointees and/or representatives?

Whatever the design choices that were made, the new bodies in Canada have been created by a universal move to garner *up* some of the more informal power of providers (such as individual hospital and community boards and individual practitioners), while devolving *down* some of the formal power and authority of provincial governments. Thus some centralization of highly fragmented and overly decentralized control has been combined with some decentralization of provincial power to form the most radical reform of the organizational structure of medicare since its inception 25 years ago.

But just how significant is this devolution of authority? Should we really consider all these new regional and local bodies to have true devolved *authority*? Anne Mills, in her exploration of decentralization of health services for the World Health Organization, makes some useful distinctions between the "de-somethings":

- *Deconcentration:* spatial redistribution of administrative authority to local offices of the central government.

- *Decentralization:* transfer to a local authority of some decisionmaking within a significantly constraining set of centrally-determined guidelines and standards.

- *Devolution:* transfer to a local authority of significant decisionmaking with only broad principles determined by central government.

Although it is almost certainly the case that the newly created regional and local bodies in Canada's provinces are arrayed across this entire "de-something" spectrum it is only partly their formal design that will determine this status. Perhaps at least as important is the discretionary interpretation and application of the formal rules by both the new body and its overseer province. For, as Robert Putnam states, devolution of authority is an ongoing negotiation:

> Devolution is inevitably a bargaining process, not simply a juridical act. The legal and constitutional framework (controls, delegated power, personnel patterns and so on), and finances are both key resources in today's game and outcomes of earlier and ongoing games. As seen by regional leaders, the central authorities' main bargaining chips are control of funds and control of formal authority — the pocketbook and the rulebook.

Therefore, just where a province's local or regional bodies lie on this de-something spectrum will, to a significant degree, depend upon the attitude and approach of the local board — their willingness to grab the power and run with it until they are stopped — and the attitude of the provincial government — their tolerance, for instance, of local boards that diverge from the central objectives of cost containment, health outcomes, and so on, as well as their willingness to allow significant variations in service delivery patterns to emerge across their province in the name of "local preferences."

A BRIEF HISTORY OF MEDICARE

To better understand this new site of potential conflict in Canada's health-care system, between provincial governments and local or regional boards, a brief detour into the history of medicare is called for (see Figures 1 to 3).

Before World War II the relationship between providers of health care and the population could be characterized as direct — dollars flowed directly from patients to providers in return for services (Figure 1). After the war, starting with hospital care, and progressing through physicians' services, home care, nursing homes and (for some segments of the population) drugs, this relationship became far more indirect. The dollars flowed via taxation, payroll and premium systems to federal and provincial governments, who in turn paid through a variety of arrangements to the various providers in return for the delivery of services to the population (Figure 2). Many have commented on the "public payment, private practice" nature of this relationship that essentially placed the provincial governments in the role of fiscal transfer station between taxpayers and providers. The consequent absence of management mechanisms that might attain cost containment, improved health outcomes, flexibility and responsiveness, and integration and coordination was another of the common themes in the provincial task forces and reports

Post-1990 the enchantment with devolved authority has imposed itself on this historical configuration (Figure 3). Devolved authorities are, therefore, expected to not only flow *dollars* to providers and providing institutions, but also to impose some management on "the system." A key question is what will be the biggest influence on the management choices of a local or regional board — the input of dollars from its provincial government or the input of "needs and wants" from its community? If the dollar inputs predominate then the devolved board becomes little more than a central enforcer located in the community (deconcentration); if the needs and wants of the community predominate then the board acts as a "local mirror" which may not reflect all that is congruent with central provincial government objectives.

Figure 1: The Health-Care "System" pre-1945

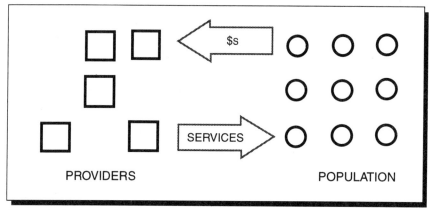

Source: Author's compilation.

Figure 2: The Health-Care "System" 1945-1990

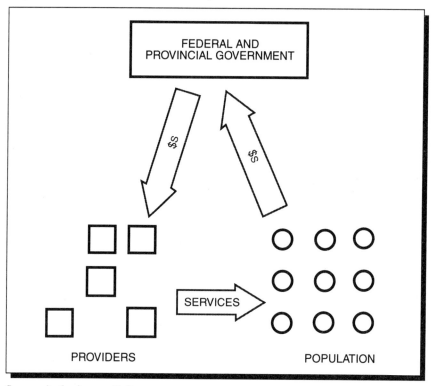

Source: Author's compilation.

Figure 3: The Health-Care "System" 1990

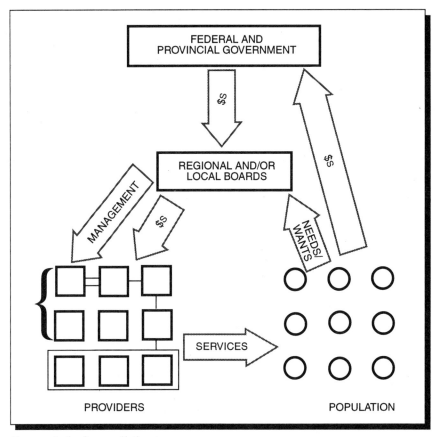

Source: Author's compilation.

THE "LOCAL MIRROR" VERSUS
"CENTRAL ENFORCER" CONTINUUM

Representation on the local or regional boards is obviously a major deter-
minant of where on the continuum between "central enforcer" and "local
mirror" each devolved authority will lie. As Putnam noted, however, it is
likely to be an ongoing and evolving negotiation with no static endpoint.
Nevertheless, the attitudes and perceived roles of current board members
may give us some clues to at least the direction in which the boards are

heading. To obtain these clues we are surveying the devolved authority board members in five provinces — British Columbia, Alberta, Saskatchewan, Nova Scotia, and Prince Edward Island. There are 76 boards in these provinces (excluding the community councils in British Columbia) and to date we have obtained cooperation from 57, refusal to participate from four, and we are "in negotiation" ourselves with the remaining 15. We have some interim results based on the 32-percent response rate from the participating boards as of May 1995. I would caution that these are *Interim* results, and may change once we have obtained our full response rate later in the summer with appropriate reminders and additional recruitment efforts.

Overall, the board members are relatively experienced with less than a third having no previous board appointments. Both their educational and income levels are "above average," and they are evenly divided between men and women. They are also a very keen lot, giving an average of 37 hours per month of volunteer time to their board activities. About 70 percent felt that their training and orientation to the task were adequate or excellent and that they had enough information to make good decisions.

Turning to the questions of more direct relevance to the potential "central enforcer" versus "local mirror" conflict, we found that they overwhelmingly (72 percent) identified local citizens as the group to which they felt most accountable (rather than the minister of health, the Ministry of Health, the provincial taxpayers, or the local group they represent). Members from the more mature boards in Saskatchewan and Alberta were more likely to feel restricted by rules laid down by their provincial government than members from the newer boards in British Columbia and Nova Scotia (500 feeling restricted in the former provinces and 30 percent in the latter). These results are suggestive of boards trying to play more of a local mirror role than being central enforcers.

Nevertheless, when the board members were asked whether they would vote for a decision that they personally felt was correct but that was opposed by the majority in their community, more than 80 percent replied that they would vote their personal view in such circumstances. Furthermore, although they *generally* felt that they had enough information to make good decisions, less than 30 percent felt that they had adequate information about local citizen preferences. Thus, the tension between the central enforcer and local mirror roles is already showing through, even though there appears to be a well-intentioned goal of being more the local mirror.

A widespread concern expressed by these board members, all of whom are currently appointees, are the plans of most of these provinces to move to fully or partially elected boards. Most of the concern centres on either the potential for the boards to become captured by single-interest groups or the likely preponderance of what respondents often called "representational politics" i.e., that elected individuals will feel accountable to identifiable interest or geographic groups rather than to local citizens in general. The irony is, of course, that these comments in opposition to elected representation, or "democracy" as we term it, are being expressed by members of bodies that provincial governments claim are the new structures "democratizing" the health-care system!

CONCLUSIONS

The emergence of devolved authorities in Canada is the latest health policy panacea, designed to achieve the long-sought objective of improved management. "Devolved command and control" appears to be a uniquely Canadian solution to this management dilemma, bucking the international trend to the use of regulated markets and competition between either payers or providers.

However, as a number of recent reports on devolution have pointed out (including the report by one of this conference's sponsors — the CMA), there is little or no prior research or evaluation to reassure us that devolving authority is likely to achieve the provincial governments' objectives of cost containment, improved health outcomes, more responsiveness and flexibility, and better integration and coordination. Indeed, there *is* some evidence to suggest that equity, in the sense of comparable services being available to comparable populations, might be a concern as local bodies pursue quite different interpretations of their mandate. In this light, our highly publicized concerns about interprovincial equity under the guise of a renewed *Canada Health Act* debate might be diverting attention from the potentially far more significant source of equity concern — over 100 devolved authorities each pursuing separate visions of medicare under varying degrees of provincial "control" and with varying degrees of vigour in their attempts to challenge this control in the name of being a mirror for local citizens' needs and wants.

It would appear imperative, therefore, to evaluate the evolution of devolved authorities and their performance, not only to track whether they are indeed achieving the objectives set for them by provincial governments, but also to monitor the extent to which they become the site and focus of medicare's inevitable conflicts. The old conflicts between provincial governments and providers with a relatively transparent self-interest, may be replaced by a far more challenging conflict in which provincial governments are confronted by devolved authorities cloaked in the protection of "mirroring local needs and wants," and armed with the imprimatur of elected status. The more effective and vigorous the devolved authority becomes in achieving the goal of better reflecting local needs, then the more likely they are to come into conflict with some provincial government vision of needs. If this turns out to be the case, then the associations and various lobbying arms of the major historic interest-groups (providers, providing institutions, patient and "disease-specific" groups, and corporate interests such as the pharmaceutical sector) face a major challenge themselves. They will have to learn to adapt to directing their efforts not at just ten provincial government sites, but at potentially more than 100 local devolved authorities, each with very different characteristics. This appears to be a challenge fit for the millennium, and certainly grist for much policy analysis!

Note

[1] It is interesting to note, however, that no provinces (indeed, few international jurisdictions) have as yet included the budget for physicians' services within the remit of the devolved authorities. This is interesting in light of the declared objective of "integration and coordination" — the integration of primary care, for instance, in the absence of any fiscal say over primary care Physicians will require particular creativity.

5

Accountability and Regionalization

Richard Fraser

INTRODUCTION

This paper will cover the important issues of accountability and regionalization. I plan to discuss the following areas: the definitions of accountability; the "what" and "who" of accountability; the "what" and "who" of liability; the "how" of accountability; and the importance of relationship. My conclusions will follow.

DEFINITIONS OF ACCOUNTABILITY (LIABILITY)

The Dictionary of Canadian Law defines *accountable* in two words — "liable and responsible." It defines *liability* as "the situation in which one is potentially or actually subject to some obligation," and *responsible* is defined as "see person."

Black's Law Dictionary (U.S.) defines *accountability* as "state of being responsible or answerable. See also liability." In Black's, the word liability occupies one and one-half columns and commences by stating "the word is a broad legal term." It goes on to state that liability is a "condition which creates a duty to perform an act immediately or in the future ... duty which must at least eventually be performed ... the state of one who is bound in law and justice to do something which may be enforced by action."

Black's goes on to define responsibility as "the state of being answerable for an obligation, and includes judgment, skill and ability and capacity."

The definition of accountability I like best relates to a person and is found in the Dictionary of Canadian Law. It defines the term "Responsible Medical Officer" as "the physician or one to whom responsibility for the *care* and treatment of an individual patient has been assigned"(emphasis added).

Therefore, for our purposes in discussing regionalization, it seems reasonable to suggest that a regional authority is the authority to whom responsibility for the *care* and treatment of patient populations, which includes patients, has been assigned. We should remember the importance of the definition of responsibility, which includes judgement, skill and ability and capacity.

I realize that this definition of accountability is somewhat narrow and perhaps traditional, but I think it gets us back to the important basics of what health authorities and providers are fundamentally responsible for. Therefore, regional authorities have accountability for system design and the provision of appropriate patient care. If they fail in these tasks through inappropriate system design or the provision of negligent care, they may well be liable.

Accountability and liability are simply the flip-side of the same coin. You cannot have accountability without liability and you cannot have liability without accountability. In fact, if you want to be truly accountable you should expect and appreciate the fact of liability. Putting it another way, accountability without any fear or concern for consequences is likely not accountability at all.

As a result, I believe accountability in the context of regionalization provides the following answers to our next two questions:

- Accountability for what — system design, care and treatment
- Accountability for who — regional populations that include individual people.

I now wish to discuss accountability for what and to who in a different context.

THE WHAT AND WHO OF ACCOUNTABILITY

Much good work has been done in Ontario concerning devolution of authority. Accountability and regionalization were included as topics for discussion in a recently held roundtable sponsored by the Project Team on Health Reform of the Ontario Premier's Council in May 1995. The roundtable was a natural evolution itself from a document entitled "A Framework for Evaluating Devolution," prepared for the Premier's Council on Health, Well-being and Social Justice. At the outset, this document stated:

> Devolution of health and social services involves the transfer of greater control and decision-making for some or all of the planning, funding, management, revenue generation and delivery functions. The degree of devolution lies along a continuum between full central control and full local/regional control.

Power may be devolved up or down. Power may devolve down from a provincial government to a regional authority and may devolve up to a regional authority from traditional hospital boards or other community providers. The document, "A Framework for Evaluating Devolution" looks at the devolution of *scope* (the what or care); *function* (the how or systems) and *authority* (financial) in assessing devolution.

In terms of analyzing *function,* Exhibit 7 of the document describes seven devolved systems functions as: planning, resource allocation, policy development, standard setting, coordination, evaluation, and delivery.

Therefore, in a hypothetical provincial regionalization devolution, we could find that such things as planning and resource allocation would be devolved down from the province to the regional authority and such things as coordination and delivery could be devolved up from hospital boards to the regional authority. Provincial governments could retain policy development, standard setting, and evaluation.

This devolution down and up results in the marriage of policy and operational functions which result in significant accountability and liability accruing to a regional authority for the design and provision of patient care to regional populations. (See Figure 1)

Figure 1: Devolution of Accountabilty

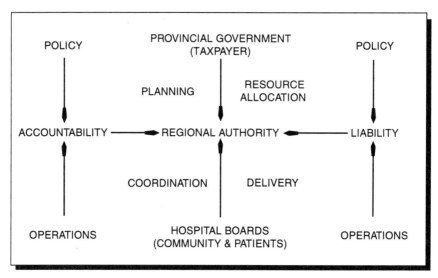

Source: Author's compilation.

THE "WHAT" AND "WHO" OF LIABILITY

The marriage of policy and operational functions results in accountability/ liability of regional authorities. It also answers the question of who do we sue. Issues concerning improper system design and provision of negligent care will surely fall at the feet of regional authorities.

The fact that regional authorities will likely be held liable for inadequate system design and negligent provision of care will be of some comfort to health-care providers who continually feel that they are in a "catch-22" situation of being required to provide health-care services when they feel they do not have proper resources.

Hopefully, this understanding of accountability/liability will allow all concerned to work cooperatively together to create the best system within existing financial resources.

The issue of resource allocation is an important one. Raisa Deber has written of the need to establish a process for determining what is medically necessary. She has concerns about a simple serial listing of services. It may be that the process should be continuing. Examination of process formed a significant part of the recommendations of a task force for the Canadian Bar Association entitled, "What's Law Got To Do With It — Health Reform in Canada" (Appendix). Included in the recommendations is a reference to practice standards.

When regional health-care practice standards are developed, they may facilitate the provision of appropriate levels and types of services. This will be very important in many different areas.

Areas of Potential Concern

What are some of the important areas that practice standards could cover, especially as they relate to the issue of prevention of liability and therefore the fulfilment of accountability? From my experience, the following areas may well be of importance: (i) downsizing of acute care; (ii) importance of emergency care; (iii) movement of patients; (iv)importance of emergency transport; (v) labour and employment relations — severance payments and retraining; (vi) health workforce rebalancing issues — multi-skilling; (vii) long-term care, including seniors; (viii) medical staff relations; (ix) new organizational structures — life without middle managers; (x) consolidation and reduction of corporate services; (xi) out-sourcing/contracting-out; and (xii) regional authority, vision and values.

Litigation Activity

In a regionalized system, will the foregoing areas that are impacted by reduction, restructuring, and reform result in increased litigation? I believe the answer is *yes*. My reasons are as follows:

- planning considerations, formerly made by provincial governments and considered policy, will no longer be clothed with legal immunity when they are made at a regional level.

- the marriage of accountability and liability in regional authorities.

- high expectations of Canadians for their health-care system.

- a greater awareness by Canadians of their rights and responsibilities concerning health care.

- reduction, restructuring, and reform that is not done through an open and inclusive process.

- reduction, restructuring, and reform that impairs effective working relationships among health-care providers
- groups of people losing services or having services reduced that were formerly covered by the health-care system, e.g., seniors.
- new standards not being developed in time to coincide with the introduction of new patien-care systems.
- conflicted care givers who may become more active in confronting decisionmakers and talking about their concerns (and being expert witnesses).
- the development by the courts of the fiduciary relationship between health-care providers and patients.

Courts will continue to focus on appropriate standards for patient care and whether there has been a breach of these standards resulting in injury to the patient. Cost containment issues will be raised and the courts will be required to respond to these arguments.

The courts have always responded to issues of medical malpractice, so they should be able in the future to deal with challenges resulting from regionalization as they occur. If governments regard the litigation process and court decisions as being counterproductive to the implementation of government policy, then we will see an attempt by governments to avoid liability including the institution of no-fault insurance programs.

Preventative Measures

As a result of the foregoing, when examining accountability-liability issues arising from regionalization, it may be helpful to seek answers to the following questions: Has there been a proper planning process? In particular, was the actual plan, its implementation and timetable reasonable? Were cost containment measures implemented in an arbitrary or unreasonable fashion? Were cost containment measures too severe? Is the need for change based upon true economic necessity? Was there proper communication among the policy setters, the operational implementors, the providers and the patients, to ensure that the plan was successfully implemented? What were the former standards of care and how were they monitored? What are the new standards of care and how will they be monitored? Are the new standards sufficient to maintain proper patient care and how can that be determined? Did leadership facilitate cooperation?

I would now like to examine the very important issue of process and relationship.

THE "HOW" OF ACCOUNTABILITY

From my experiences with the Canadian Bar Association task force on health care and my work in Alberta during the process of regionalization, I believe that the *how* or the *process* may be the most important issue to review in accountability and regionalization. The how will necessarily include what you are prepared to do in implementing regionalization. As John Carver describes the issue of setting values, it is the things that you are not prepared to do that may clearly define what you are prepared to do to achieve an end result. Does the end justify the means? Understanding, articulating, and following values is critical for successful health-care reform.

Command and Control

For the present, I believe that the how of regionalization has been and likely will continue to be command and control. This is to be contrasted with cooperation and true consultation. Command and control starts in legislation and works its way down through the health-care system often by regulation and through the use of the adversarial process. This can cause immense frustration to people working in the health-care system (who normally work together) and to members of the public who become concerned about whether or not the new system will adequately meet their needs.

Jonathan Lomas has noted that the Canadian health system has been unique in the world and that Canada has evolved a system of command and control going up and down. He noted that devolution is a bargaining process. I believe that this bargaining process can easily become adversarial in nature in which there are truly winners and losers. He also noted the importance of the central enforcer (provincial government) applying pressure to a regional authority from above and from below, pressure exerted by the community or local mirror. This analysis also fits with my earlier comments concerning the marriage of accountability and liability.

David Peterson made the important point that for political leaders, dealing with what Bob Evans describes as the issue from hell, you can either buy it (build hospitals) or have a crisis (close hospitals). How true this has been in my own province of Alberta! The golden rule of spending (he or she who controls the gold, rules) and the fear created from a supposed crisis are powerful controllers.

Marie Fortier talked about federal levers of power being criminal law (certainly scary); spending powers (buying it); and peace, order and good government (emergency powers used in a crisis). Again, these are powerful controllers.

Alan Maynard reminded us that whether you are in a private or a public system, there are always regulations. In the public system, the regulation is mainly done by government. In the United States, this regulation is done to a very large extent by the legal system and the courts.

The difficulty with the command and control paradigm for achieving accountability, especially when the adversarial process is also used, is that the fundamental concern of health-care providers in providing care can be replaced with a concern for survival. Rather than having a cooperative community seeking to maximize care, we can find ourselves in an adversarial setting where people become concerned with self-interest.

Cooperation and Team Work

John Malcom described a process of focusing on only what you own, making no excuses and having the public interest paramount. Paul LaMarche stated that regionalization can allow a healthy democratic forum for debate. It identifies community health needs and attempts to get a buy-in from all participants. This requires real work.

It is because of these concerns that it is always important to focus on vision and mission. For example, the Capital Health Authority in the Edmonton region has, as its vision for health: individuals, families, and communities working together to promote and achieve improved health and quality health services. Its mission is to work in partnership with the community to create and maintain an integrated, accessible, and affordable health system with quality client services as the focus; and improved health and well-being our constant standard.

The Importance of Values

Vision and mission are critical but must also be supported by values. The values allow and protect the process and the how. Leaders must be prepared to die, at least in an organizational sense, for these values.

Recently I observed a mission-driven organization with true cooperation, collaboration, and team work. I visited the MDS Health Group Limited Regional Laboratory in Toronto. Ron Yamada acted as our guide and was quickly replaced with one employee after another. I observed true empowerment of individuals, whether in their own right or as members of a team, dealing with day-to-day and long-term issues. Values were alive and well.

The importance of the *how* or *process* to a health-care system cannot be underestimated. It is not underestimated in the best of the best in private industry. It can be summarized in a powerful passage from David Whyte's book, *The Heart Aroused*:

> Trying to run complex companies, big or small, by imperial command, from the top down, may be *the* single most unnecessary burden carried by any corporate manager. Attempting something that is doomed to fail, they produce a manual of required responses covering all eventualities. Doing this, the system they are forced to employ becomes Byzantine and cumbersome. It also carries an implicit lack of trust in the essential elements of the system — people. Not only that, but hierarchal systems based on power emanating from the top cannot plan for the wild efflorescence of impossible events that we call daily life. They are continually immobilized by the changing nature of reality. They lack robustness, adaptability, and in computer simulations with the command "form a flock," instead of flowing lifelike around obstacles, the mass of individual elements moves in the jerky mannerisms of a B-movie dinosaur.

Powerful and poetic statements. I believe they are true. I have always been fascinated that in times of true emergencies, whether by fire or flood, that normal rules of command and control give way to self-organization, teamwork, and collaboration. Why are we always constantly amazed at how much we care for one another and how well we work together without either command and control or adversarial structures in place?

Perhaps the importance of relationship is at play.

THE IMPORTANCE OF RELATIONSHIP

Beyond the how and process implications for system reform, the command and control and adversarial paradigms carry with them implicit rejection of mutually supportive relationships. They do not encourage Malcolm Anderson's "everyone at the table" or Paul LaMarche's "democratic forum for debate." A failure to recognize the harmful effects of these paradigms can have long lasting effects on a health-care system.

It is perhaps easier to view these relationships in concrete terms. One important relationship in the health-care system is the relationship between physicians and nurses. A recent proposal by the Alberta Medical Association entitled "Alternative Remuneration for Primary Care: Fee for Comprehensive Care Option" states:

> Others, notably some health care economists and nurses, are pursuing their own agendas. For them, eliminating Fee For Service is only one step in changing the role and contributions of physicians. The Alberta Association of Registered Nurses continues to press for all physicians to be paid by salary and has lobbied the regional health authorities to implement nurse-directed primary care models. (p. 3)

In a recent issue of the *Medical Post*, Dr. Augustin Roy, past president and secretary-general of the Collège des médecins du Quebec, warned that physicians will pay the price for not being vigilant in guarding their territory. He stated that: "It is up to physicians to play their role ... The nurses want to improve their status and the money that comes with it. They are hungry, and we are not hungry any more. We will be very sorry for that in 10 or 20 years from now. We don't seem to realize we will suffer."

The foregoing comments may result from unique local conditions but nevertheless should be contrasted with comments found in the Ontario College of Family Physicians Document entitled "Bringing the Pieces Together: Planning for Future Health Care." Under the heading "Nurse and Family Physician Health Care Teams" it says:

> For years, family physicians have worked effectively and efficiently with nurses and nurse practitioners, especially those with skills training in family medicine. In many instances across the province they work closely as a team to provide a wide range of services, thereby improving opportunities for patient contact, education and counselling. Such teamwork generally

represents a more efficient use of resources and expertise. Unfortunately our current system is not conducive to encouraging this teamwork, largely as a result of the current fee reimbursement mechanisms. (p. 17)

It is important to note that a funding mechanism can act as a controller that impairs relationships. Ask yourself as well, how much physicians are paid for talking with patients. I have always believed that words do have consequences. They can build or destroy relationships.

CONCLUDING COMMENTS

> "The way through the world
> is more difficult to find than the way beyond it."
>
> Wallace Stevens
> Reply to Papini

From my experience and particularly what has occurred in Alberta, I believe that we are not dealing with a metaphor of "How many roads ...?" but more likely should be using the metaphor "How many rivers...?" I believe there are likely two rivers, both with powerful currents.

One river is a result of command and control and adversarial streams, whereas the other river is fed from well springs of respect for diversity, flexibility, and interdependence. Both rivers at the edge are relatively calm, become increasingly turbulent further out and then once in the centre, individuals and populations are swept away on very strong currents that make it difficult, if not impossible, for them to ever return to the same place.

In health care, it is a good idea to study the rivers carefully. Look for the values — your paddles. Do the values encourage cooperation or invite competition?

Unfortunately, in Alberta, although we started off from a solid pier with an excellent document entitled, "Starting Points," we quickly became lost in the currents because values had not been established, or values were not clearly articulated and followed. Not everyone was in the canoe at the start. In any event, it was easy to make the mistake of turning the canoe in midstream — or maybe it turned itself because we had no paddles. Unfortunately, canoes often come to harm when turned 180° in rapids.

When health-care providers are thrown into a command and control and adversarial setting, they can easily become concerned with self-preservation. That is not their fault but the fault of leadership. Leadership at all levels. Especially leadership without values.

Many thought-provoking questions have been raised in this volume. From Jonathan Lomas wondering about the paradox of decentralization in an already fragmented delivery system to Raisa Deber asking why we are drawing boundaries when information technology is decentralizing human interaction.

Hopefully these and many other thoughtful questions will be asked before, during and after we move onto the river.

Appendix
The Canadian Bar Association
Task Force Report

"What's Law Got to Do with It?"
Health Care Reform in Canada

August 1994

SUMMARY OF CONCLUSIONS AND RECOMMENDATIONS

In this report, the Task Force on Health Care has attempted to survey the legal issues raised by changes to the health care system in Canada. We have examined the possibility of a right to health care protected by the Charter, and the scope of the entitlement to health care in the absence of such a right. We have reviewed the means by which the entitlement to health care may be enforced, both by government and by the individual. Finally, we have looked at the process used to make decisions regarding health care resource allocation at the federal, provincial and institutional levels and given special consideration to the impact of cost constraints on the relationship between the patient and the health care provider.

The goal of the Task Force in preparing this report was first to clarify the relevance of law to the study of health care delivery and health care reform and secondly, to provide an overview of the issues involved. The Task Force regards this report not as an exhaustive study of these issues, but as a means of providing a legal perspective to the public debate on health care reform. It is our hope that the report will serve as a springboard for further study of the issues raised both by lawyers and non-lawyers.

1. While the public health care system has historically been based on an insurance model, this model does not accurately reflect the current reality of health care delivery.

RECOMMENDATION: Use of the insurance model as the basis for the public health care system should be reviewed.

2. The federal government has reduced its percentage contribution to the provinces for health care over the last decade.

    While health care is a matter of provincial jurisdiction, there is a federal role in the health care through areas of specific federal power, such as the spending power, the national concern doctrine, immigration (medical screening) and criminal law (drug control)

    There is no right to health care under the *Charter of Rights and Freedoms.*

    Notwithstanding the above, there is a general expectation among the Canadian public that there is a right to health care. As a result, there is a gap between the lack of a right to health care and the expectation by the public.

    There is an express or implied right to health insurance under provincial health insurance acts, but this does not constitute a right to health care because there is no guarantee of content of health insurance (i.e., provinces may deinsure services as they choose). Further, there is no guarantee of procedural fairness in how insured services are selected or delisted (deinsured).

    Provinces are currently reducing or deinsuring services without reference to clearly articulated criteria, and without a well-defined process.

    RECOMMENDATION: Those provinces which do not have a legislated right to health care should define and legislate such a right.

3. The terms "medically necessary" and "medically required" have not been statutorily defined.

    RECOMMENDATION: Each province and territory and the federal government should enact a definition of the term "medically necessary," which would apply equally to the term "medically required."

RECOMMENDATION: Explicit criteria should be used to define this term, regardless of whether the government enacting the definition has legislated a right to health care.

RECOMMENDATION: The definition of "medically necessary" should be arrived at through an open process of cooperation and negotiation among the federal and provincial governments, to achieve uniformity to the greatest possible extent.

RECOMMENDATION: To define a right to health care, each province and territory should

i)   express a commitment to the principles underlying this right, which include the right to informed consent, the right to respect for individual autonomy and to procedural protection for the equitable distribution of health care resources, regardless of region, socioeconomic status or personal attributes;

ii) in determining which services will be provided, set out the criteria to be used, such as clinical practice standards, assessment of outcomes effectiveness, economic constraints and ethical priority-setting;

iii) establish an open process of consultation with all health care providers, consumer representatives and others for defining the right to health care. The public should be aware of the alternatives under consideration.

4.   Although there is no right to health care under the Charter, it does provide procedural protection for the equitable distribution of health care benefits.

Payment from both a provincial health plan and a resident of a province or territory for insured services constitutes a violation of the *Canada Health Act*.

RECOMMENDATION: There should be an open process of study, consultation and debate to clearly define the role of public health care and whether this is a role for private health care, and if there is, its extent, and to deal specifically with any overlap or duplication.

RECOMMENDATION: The decision to reduce or to deinsure health care services should be accomplished through a fair, open and consultative process.

RECOMMENDATION: Procedural fairness in the allocation of resources should be implemented at the institutional/facility level (e.g., the development of waiting lists).

RECOMMENDATION: Informed consent includes the right to disclosure of resource constraints which will affect treatment. This principle may be effected either through legislation or through common law.

PRACTICAL CONSIDERATIONS

6

International Experience with Decentralization and Regionalization

Northern Europe

Raisa Deber

How is regionalization progressing in Northern Europe? That is the question I plan to address here. However, any attempt to answer it must bear two points in mind.

First, although we keep using the terms synonymously, regionalization is not the same thing as decentralization. Regionalization represents the movement of power or authority to some intermediate level; it should be termed decentralization only if that power had formerly rested at a higher level (e.g., the province). If power had previously been at the local or institutional level, regionalization can instead be an example of centralization. As some have recognized, in the Canadian context, many "regional reforms" imply shifting power from individual local institutions (such as hospitals) upwards to new intermediate levels of authority (such as regional boards), with the added bonus to provincial governments of the likelihood of greater ability to control the smaller number of organizations that result (Ontario 1995).

Second, what is going on in most European countries does not really fit under the "regionalization" rubric. In Canada, we are operating with one particular view about how health systems should operate, which is not necessarily shared by other countries. In that connection, it may be helpful to give a brief description of the framework that we have been using to look at international health systems. The framework arises from some work I did with Lynn Curry, Orvil Adams, and George Pink for Health Canada (Adams *et al.* 1992; Deber *et al.* 1994, 76-91), but has subsequently been undergoing modification to look at issues of the public-private mix.

The framework is built on three dimensions: financing (how the money is raised), delivery (how services are provided), and allocation (the basis on which funds are allotted to service providers).

It begins by recognizing that both financing and delivery have public and private components.

Table 1: Examples of Health-Care Systems, Classified by Financing and Delivery

Delivery	Financing	
	Public	Private
Public	National Health Service	—
Private	Public Insurance System	Private Insurance System

Source: Author's compilation.

Table 1 thus leads to three broad categories of health-care systems. In the public financing-public delivery cell are the National Health Services, in which service providers are civil servants. This model used to exist in Scandinavia, many Eastern block countries, and the UK, but is currently under considerable reform pressure to introduce more client sensitivity (Deber *et al.* 1994). In the private financing-private delivery is the private insurance system, or idealized US system (although in actuality the public sector plays a considerable role in financing such systems — both directly and through subsidies). The public financing-private delivery cell contains two variants: the tax-based insurance characteristic of Canada, and the heavily regulated sickness funds characteristic of the "Bismarck"-influenced systems in Germany or the Netherlands.

My own reading of the international evidence is that, for medically required services, the best approach is public financing, both because monopsony control over providers gives superior cost control, and because a single source of funding avoids what is variously referred to as "cream skimming," "cherry picking," or "picking the raisins" — that is, insurers profiting by refusing to insure those at higher risk (Reinhardt 1992; Evans 1990). However, the superiority of public control, in my view, does not hold for delivery. There is considerable literature suggesting that public delivery often means less client responsiveness (Starr 1989; Bendick 1989), and the "reinventing government" movement is crafted to try to introduce incentives for cost-efficiency and quality (Reinhardt 1992). In that connection, it is important to recognize that public and private both contain many levels. Public can imply national, state/provincial, regional, or local activities, whereas private can encompass activities by charitable not-for-profit (by either volunteer or paid workers), small business-entrepreneurial or for-profit corporate organizations, as well as by individuals and their families. Particular caution must be exercised for activities for which it is difficult to measure outcomes and design performance indicators. Thus, the evidence appears to suggest that economic efficiencies may arise from privatizing the delivery of services with easily-specified quality measurements (e.g., garbage collection) to for-profit firms, but that one would be less sanguine in encouraging for-profit health care or social services; not-for-profit organizations appear to have a superior record (Bendick 1989).

It is accordingly important to recognize that different combinations of public and private apply to different sectors within health care, as well as to different countries. For example, the Canadian system indeed can be categorized as public financing and private delivery for insured medical and hospital services. However, a considerable portion of such sectors as rehabilitation, long-term care, and out-patient pharmaceuticals is privately financed and privately delivered. (Fairly predictably, unless regulated by a funder with strong market power, these sectors have also given rise to cost escalation and equity concerns.)

Understanding European reforms must therefore begin with what those countries are evolving from and what they wish to accomplish. For example, the UK and Scandinavia had represented the mix of public financing and public delivery which our framework would suggest gave fairly good cost control, good equity, but fairly poor client responsiveness; one would expect reforms to address these concerns. In contrast, Germany and the Netherlands have relied upon sickness funds for financing, and combined this with private delivery. Our framework would predict that the pluralistic array would give rise to a certain degree of risk-shifting across insurers, and to cost-control problems from the absence of monopsony, and to expect this to be a key focus of reforms in those systems. Indeed, it is noteworthy that the sickness funds are heavily regulated and tend to cooperate, to the extent that they operate as quasi-single source payers.

The next set of issues relates to how money is allocated to providers. We have adapted the following typology from Richard Saltman, who has arrayed allocation mechanisms on a continuum from "patient follows money" to "money follows patient."

Table 2: Allocation Models for Publicly-Financed Services

Clients Follow Money		Money Follows Clients		
Centrally planned models	Regionally planned models	Managed competition	Public competition	Pure market

Source: Author's compilation.

The planned end of the continuum gives stronger cost control (i.e., organizations are allocated global budgets with which to provide services, and patients have to go where those services are offered). The market end gives greater client responsiveness (i.e., organizations are allocated money only if they attract patients). The mechanisms in the centre represent various — largely untested and unevaluated — attempts to get the advantages, and not the disadvantages, of both. We postulate that one cannot alter either financing or delivery without making some corresponding changes to allocation.

Against this background, I will present my understanding of what has been happening, based upon recent visits to Sweden and the Netherlands and a limited use of the literature; given the limitations of understanding inherent in such international visits and the rapidity of change, these remarks should be treated with the appropriate cautions.

Table 3:   Sweden — Proposed Reforms

Aspect	Current	Proposed Changes
Financing	Public • county council (with some revenue sharing)	None
Delivery	Public • county council	"Privatize" to mediating structures
Allocation	Regionally planned	Public competition

Source: Author's compilation.

Sweden has not been trying to change from public financing; indeed, the virtually unanimous advice they received from the international expert panels they consulted as part of their reexamination of their system was that they should not touch financing. Instead, they have been trying to modify delivery to shorten waiting lists, put more emphasis on primary care, and encourage responsiveness (Sweden Expert Group 1993; Maynard 1993; Culyer 1991; Culyer et al. 1991; Deber 1993; Rehnberg 1994; Hakansson 1994; Diderichsen 1993; Saltman 1990; Berleen et al. 1992; Saltman and van Otter 1992; Ham 1992). In that sense, they are "privatizing" delivery by shifting providers away from their former status as employees of the county councils. In some places, this direction is being resisted by county councils who enjoyed micro-managing health-care delivery (to the extent that, we were informed, some county councillors had seen it as their responsibility to check hospital inventories and personally count the sheets). This means some pressure to change allocation to reward those who can attract clients, or meet other goals, such as reducing waiting lists. The experiments with public competition in some Swedish counties have been well described by Saltman and von Otter (Saltman and von Otter 1992).

Table 4: Netherlands — Proposed Reforms

Aspect	Current	Proposed Changes
Financing	Mixed: public and private • sickness funds	Shift from employers to families, nation
Delivery	Private	No change
Allocation	Pure market	Managed competition

Source: Author's compilation.

In contrast, the Netherlands and Germany appeared to be quite happy with their form of delivery, but were concerned because so much of the financing was borne by employers; they saw the resulting payroll taxes as job killers. Accordingly, they were trying to move financing away from payroll taxes — even if it meant a greater private role and more costs — but also using regulation to cap costs (e.g., around money paid to physicians, or for drugs). In the Netherlands, the reforms concentrated on financing — with various proposals about how to match public and private sickness funds, who would be covered by each, and for what services. This in turn has led to some modifications on allocation to try to improve cost control — including Enthoven-type proposals in the Netherlands for a "purchaser-provider split" (Osborne and Gaebler 1992). It is noteworthy, however, that as of when I was there, sickness funds were not using their power to direct contracts to low bidders. Sickness funds continued to sign up "all willing providers," and those I spoke with claimed that it would not be seen as appropriate to limit choice of provider. So the current Dutch reform plans bear very little resemblance to that which had been proposed for the US under the rubric of "managed competition," which is premised on the idea of competition driving the less competitive providers out of business.

What is going on in Canada?

Table 5: Canada — Proposed Reforms

Aspect	Current	Proposed Changes
Financing	Public • federal/provincial	Shares
Delivery	Private • non profit (hospitals) and small businesses (mds)	Publicize to regional boards
Allocation	Pure market	Regionally planned

Source: Author's compilation.

Canada's perception is that the major problems deal with cost control, particularly since few provinces have taken much advantage of monopsony control until relatively recently, along with some rigidity — which we refer to in terms of paying tribute to our agricultural heritage as "silos" — arising from the way in which we have defined spending envelopes. The Canadian reforms are accordingly trying to move away from open-ended funding, and to better coordination (Evans 1992; Hurley *et al*. 1994; Rachlis and Kusher 1989; 1994).

In our terminology, the Canadian problems would be categorized as allocation problems. However, a number of Canadian provinces are instead attempting to address them through trying to modify delivery. I could, but will not discuss some of the resulting issues. These include a number of technical and procedural issues which will have considerable effects on the outcomes of health policy — for example, how much variation is permissible, how boundaries will be set, who will decide on resource allocation, and the processes which will be used. I will just note that specific, governmental responses to these questions become necessary only because some provinces are moving to the planned end of the allocation continuum, and that using other mechanisms would make some of these questions moot.

In examining Canada through international lenses, I found it striking that we appear to be moving towards systems which Sweden, as one example, is trying to move away from. But policy is like a pendulum, as the recent Ontario election has shown. Accordingly, it may be important to conclude with an insight of the late Aaron Wildavsky — when dealing with complex policy problems, one never solves them. Instead, one replaces one set of problems with another. The mark of success is whether one prefers the new set of problems to the old set (Wildavsky 1979). In that respect, the jury remains out on all systems, and we will have to return to these questions in the future.

References

Adams, O., L. Curry and R.B. Deber. 1992. *Public and Private Health Care Financing: Literature Review and Description: Volumes 1 & 2*. Ottawa: Curry Adams & Associates.

Bendick, M. Jr. 1989. "Privatizing the Delivery of Social Welfare Services: An Ideal to Be Taken Seriously." In: *Privatization and the Welfare State*, ed. S.B. Kamerman and S.B. Kahn. Princeton, NJ: Princeton University Press. pp. 97-120.

Berleen, G., S. Hakansson, C. Rehnberg and G. Wennström. 1992. *The Reform of Health Care in Sweden*. National report to OECD. April.

Culyer, A.J. 1991. *Health Care and Health Care Finance in Sweden: The Crisis that Never Was — The Tensions that Ever Will Be*. Summary of an International Review of the Swedish Health Care System, Occasional Paper No. 33, Stockholm.

Culyer, A.J., R.G. Evans, J.-MG. von der Schulenburg, W.P. van de Ven and B.A. Weisbrod. 1991. *International Review of the Swedish Health Care System*. Occasional Paper No. 34, Stockholm.

Deber, R.B. 1993. *Reflections Concerning a Future Swedish Model for Health Care: The View from Canada*. Paper prepared for the Committee on Funding and Organisation of Health Services and Medical Care (HSU 2000). Stockholm.

Deber, R.B., O. Adams and L. Curry. 1994. "International Healthcare Systems: Models of Financing and Reimbursement." In *Proceedings of the Fifth Canadian Conference on Health Economics*, by J.A. Boan. Regina: Canadian Plains Research Center.

Diderichsen, F. 1993. "Market Reforms in Swedish Health Care: A Threat to or Salvation for the Universalistic Welfare State?" *International Journal of Health Services* 23, 1:185-88.

Evans, R.G. 1990. "Tension, Compression, and Shear: Directions, Stresses, and Outcomes of Health Care Cost Control," *Journal of Health Politics, Policy and Law* 15, 1:101-08.

_____. 1992. "Canada: The Real Issues," *Journal of Health Politics, Policy and Law* 17, 4:739-762.

Hakansson, S. 1994. "New Ways of Financing and Organizing Health Care in Sweden," *International Journal of Health Planning Management* 9:103-124.

Ham, C. 1992. "Reforming the Swedish Health Services: The International Context," *Health Policy* 21:129-41.

Hurley, J., J. Lomas and V. Bhatia. 1994. "When Tinkering Is not Enough: Provincial Reform to Manage Health Care Resources," *Canadian Public Administration* 37, 3:490-514.

Jérôme-Forget, M., J. White and J.M. Wiener, eds. 1995. *Health Care Reform Through Internal Markets: Experience and Proposals.* Ottawa: The Institute for Research on Public Policy/The Brookings Institution.

Kirkman-Liff, B.L. 1991. "Health Insurance Values and Implementation in the Netherlands and the Federal Republic of Germany," *Journal of the American Medical Association* 25, 19:2496-2502.

Laetz, T.J. and M.W. Freeman. 1995. *The Netherlands Care Sector: Balancing Marketplace Incentives with Government Regulations.* Paper distributed at the Four Country Conference on Health Care Policies and Health Care Reform in United States, Canada, Germany, The Netherlands, Amsterdam, 23-25 February.

Lapre, R.M. 1988. "A Change of Direction in the Dutch Healthcare System?" *Health Policy Quarterly* 10:21-32.

Maynard, A. 1993. *Myth and Reality in Health Care Reform: Managed Care, Internal Markets and Other Fairy Stories.* Paper prepared for the hearing by the Committee on the Funding and Organisation of Health Services and Medical Care (HSU 2000).

Okma, K.G.H. 1994. *Food for Hungry Academicians: The Issues in the Debate on Health Care Reforms in the Netherlands.* Ministry of Health, Welfare, and Sport of the Netherlands and Yale: School of Organization and Management.

_____. 1995. *Regulating the Private Insurance Market in the Netherlands.* Ministry of Health, Welfare, and Sport.

Ontario. Premier's Council Project Team on Health Reform. 1995. *Challenging Assumptions: Restructuring Health Systems Across Canada. Devolution or Dog's Breakfast.* Toronto: Ontario Premier's Council, Project Team on Health Reform.

Osborne, D.E. and T. Gaebler. 1992. *Reinventing Government: How the Entrepreneurial Spirit is Transforming the Public Sector*. Reading, MA: Addison-Wesley Publications.

Rachlis, M. and C. Kushner. 1989. *Second Opinion: What's Wrong With Canada's Health Care System and How to Fix It*. Toronto: Collins Publishing.

_____. 1994. *Strong Medicine: How to Save Canada's Health Care System*. Toronto: HarperCollins Publishers.

Rehnberg, C. 1994. *The Swedish Experience with Internal Markets*. Paper presented at the Institute for Research on Public Policy/The Brookings International Conference. Montreal. May.

Reinhardt, U.E. 1992. "The United States: Breakthroughs and Waste," *Journal of Health Politics, Policy and Law* 17, 2:637-666.

Saltman, R.B. 1990. "Competition and Reform in the Swedish Health System," *Milbank Quarterly* 68, 4:597-618.

Saltman, R.B. and C. von Otter. 1992. *Planned Markets and Public Competition: Strategic Reform in Northern European Health Systems*. Philadelphia: Open University Press.

_____. 1992. "Reforming Swedish Health Care in the 1990s: The Emerging Role of 'Public Firms'." *Health Policy* 21:143-54.

Scheerder, R.L.J.M. 1995. *Cost Containment Policy in Canada and the United States, Germany and the Netherlands*. Paper prepared for the Four Country Conference on Health Care Policies and Health Care Reform in United States, Canada, Germany and the Netherlands, Amsterdam, 23-25 February.

Starr, P. 1989. "The Meaning of Privatization." In *Privatization and the Welfare State*, ed. S.B. Kamerman and A.J. Kahn. Princeton, NJ: Princeton University Press. pp. 15-48.

Sweden Expert Group. 1993. *Three Models for Health Care Reform in Sweden*. Report from the Expert Group to the Committee on Funding and Organisation of Health Services and Medical Care, (HSU 2000). Sweden: Ministry of Health and Social Affairs.

van de Ven, W.P. 1994. *The Dutch Experience with Internal Markets*. Institute for Research on Public Policy/The Brookings International Conference, Montreal. 15-16 May.

Wildavsky, A. 1979. *Speaking Truth to Power: The Art and Craft of Policy Analysis*. Boston: Little Brown and Company.

United Kingdom

Alan Maynard

INTRODUCTION

Public policymakers have an incentive to be vague about the nature and ranking of their objectives: the absence of clarity ensures that it is much more difficult to make these decisionmakers accountable for their actions! In any economic analysis of health policy there is an emphasis on efficiency and equity. However, for the policymaker the primary concern is expenditure control, i.e., cost containment. What is the nature of the terms efficiency, equity and cost containment? And what lessons can be learned from international experience about the effective pursuit of these goals?

These goals are pursued in political frameworks with varying degrees of centralization and decentralization. A recent trend has been for politicians, often but not always of the ideological right, to de-cry centralization and advocate the redistribution of power to provinces, regions, and localities. Often this rhetoric is insincere as central politicians are unlikely to yield functions to others which reduce both their power and their capacity to garner votes to ensure reelection. However, sometimes such power is redistributed because of changes in the relative fiscal capacities of federal and provincial authorities. Such decentralization may make the achievement of equity, efficiency, and cost control across the nation less easy (i.e., in the Canadian context, it may undermine the substantive effects of the *Canada Health Act* even if its principles remain part of federal rhetoric.

COST CONTAINMENT

Uwe Reinhardt emphasized the expenditure-income identity nearly two decades ago in his essay "Table Manners at the Health Care Feast" (1978).

Households can be "robbed" of their resources by health-care financing organizations which take their money in the form of private insurance contributions, of social insurance (which is, of course, merely taxation disguised as "insurance" by politicians in a nice combination of fiscal illusion and fiscal ignorance to trick the public), of explicit taxation, and of user charges (co-payments).

These funds can be dispensed by the funders of health care who, in both public and private health-care systems, have only latterly become aware that the purchasing power they possess can be used to manipulate the behaviour of providers, that is they can act as price-makers rather than price-takers. Their funds are typically spent on purchasing care from providers in return for payments based on fee-per-item of service, capitation, and salary.

These payments create the revenue for provider agencies — they create the income and jobs of doctors, nurses, hospitals, managers, and the pharmaceutical industry. Any attempt to control health-care expenditures leads to the control of both job creation and income generation. A reform of the health-care system typically redistributes both expenditures and the jobs and incomes of providers. As a consequence, change may be unpopular!

In any consideration of cost-containment policies it is essential to remember the expenditure-income relationship. Cost controls inevitably damage the interests of suppliers who will protest using often poorly articulated arguments which infer harm to the achievement of efficiency and equity goals and the interests of patients. Such self-interested responses are also produced by effective cost-containment policies.

While the body of evidence is limited, and to some degree contentious (Wolfe and Moran) it seems that the necessary, but not sufficient, conditions for expenditure control in the health-care sector are global budget caps and "single-pipe" financing. The sufficient condition for the success of any such controls is political dedication which is often short term and related to the electoral cycle in reality. However, if the politicians want cost control, it is achievable.

Single pipe financing, usually from taxation, is needed because if there are several pipes or sources of funding, constriction of one pipe will lead to an inflation of another, for example, public expenditure control may lead to private expenditure increases which result in little net overall effect on health-care expenditure. The global budgets in places such as the United Kingdom, Sweden, and Germany have, to varying degrees, controlled the rate of growth of health-care expenditure.

User charges (co-payments) are contentious. Barer, Evans and Stoddart concluded (1994) in reviews in 1979 and 1994 that they are "misguided and cynical attempts to tax the ill and/or drive up the total cost of health care while shifting some of the burden out of government budgets." Without doubt such charges reduce utilization. To the extent that any level of utilization of health-care services is inefficient this is the product of doctors' behaviours. It is they who determine access to health-care services and the logic of charging the consumer to improve the efficiency of the providers' resource allocation decisions is absent: surely the optimal policy would be to use incentives (e.g., guidelines and financial rewards and penalties) to affect provider behaviour directly? The efficacy of user charges as a method of reducing cost inflation is unproven. Particular patient demands may be reduced by such charges but compensating demand may arise elsewhere in the system, for example, charges for primary care visits may lead to reduced use of such provision and increased use of "free" hospital emergency services. Whilst user charges are thus generally inefficient, inequitable, and do not facilitate cost control, they may be used by vote-maximizing politicians as a means by which tax burdens can be manipulated relatively (i.e., between groups) and absolutely.

Thus, if policymakers wish to achieve control over the expenditure on health care a combination of political determination, global budgets, and single-pipe finance seem likely to be effective. These lessons apply both to central government and in federal states to the provinces. If power is decentralized in such a way as to give discretion to provinces with regard to choice of funding (e.g., allowing Canadian provinces to encourage private insurance despite the provisions of the *Canada Health Act*), then cost control is likely to become more difficult (as well as having implications for equity and efficiency). It is remarkable how these lessons are ignored by policymakers worldwide but, of course, such behaviour often reflects political preferences for "diversity in funding" (i.e., private finance) which can yield voting dividends from tax reductions and other vote maximizing behaviours.

EQUITY

There are a variety of perspectives on equity in health and health care; equity in budget allocation; equity in access and use of health care; and equity in health status.

The British have used weighted capitation budget formulae for decades, unlike Canadians who, at the provincial level, are only just beginning to use such mechanisms (e.g., in Saskatchewan). Each component part of the United Kingdom has a separate formula for the allocation of hospital budgets. The one used for England is based on the work of the Resource Allocation Working Party (RAWP) and this weights population for need by using regional mortality data. This results in more resources going to these areas that kill off more of their population! A recent revision of the formula has led to a potentially radical redistribution of funding geographically because, *inter alia*, it introduces variables such as single person households and unemployment as measures of need (Peacock and Smith 1995; Carr-Hill *et al.* 1994; Smith *et al.* 1994).

The more equitable distribution of health-care resources does not necessarily create either greater equality in access to care or greater health equality. The typical patient wants access to cost-effective health care, but what he typically confronts is the clinician's uncertainty about outcomes, let alone costs, as well as a great variation in how individual doctors respond to similar clinical conditions. The small area variations in clinical activity rates, described in great detail by Wennberg (1993) in the United States, are common to all health-care systems and make the advantage of meeting the goal of access equity clearly dependent on demonstrable appropriateness and cost effectiveness.

Equity in the allocation of health-care resources and equity in access to care may have little impact on health equality. Variations in health (once called inequalities in health!) are the products of differences in genetic endowment and entitlements to resources — income, wealth, housing, education, and employment. The marginal productivity of some of these inputs to the health production process appear to exceed the benefits of health care (see e.g., Wennberg 1993; Grossman 1972).

Despite this knowledge, the dominance of ideology has led to many governments adopting policies which are predicated on the basis that sharp financial incentives are necessary to generate economic growth. Such an approach, together with "monetarist policies" which give priority to price control (i.e., low rates of inflation) at the cost of employment has resulted in increased inequalities in income and wealth (for UK data see Table 1). The effects of such inequalities on the health of particular cohorts is unlikely to be beneficial (Grossman 1972; McKeown 1974; Judge 1995).

Any equalization of financial capacity within countries and within regions or provinces may, over time, reduce inequalities in the access to health care but will not necessarily equalize health. Few jurisdictions have found an effective means to coordinate the allocation of public expenditure to maximize health as this requires the management of many public policies and, at the margin, the reallocation of resources from health care (where productivity is low) to other activities such as income redistribution. Such policies are often unpopular as they reduce the income of powerful voting groups and advantage often inarticulate minorities who are politically inactive (e.g., poor ethnic groups).

Table 1: Shares of Total Income for Each Quintile of the Income Distribution

| | | | *Percentages of Income After Housing Costs* | | | |
			1979	*1981*	*1987*	*1988/89*
Quintile	1	(Poorest)	9.6	9.1	7.6	6.9
	2		14.1	13.6	12.4	12.2
	3		18.0	17.8	16.8	17.1
	4		23.1	23.0	23.0	23.1
	5	(Richest)	35.2	36.5	40.2	40.7

Source: Jenkins, S.P. and F.A. Cowell, "Dwarfs and Giants in the 1980s: The UK Income Distribution and How It Changed." Discussion Paper 93-03. University College of Swansea, Department of Economics.

EFFICIENCY

The definition of efficiency is often confused in the health policy debate. The essential distinctions are: (i) the doctor's individual perspective: to do all that is effective for the patient; and (ii) the economists' social perspective: to do all that is cost effective for the patient.

An intervention may affect the length and quality of life of a patient but at such a high cost that it is inefficient to use it. Thus, intervention A may produce ten years of good quality life (ten quality adjusted life years or QALYs), while intervention B produces five QALYs. An effectiveness or benefit (QALY) maximizing doctor would adopt intervention A.

However, if intervention A produces ten QALYs and costs $100,000, and intervention B produces five QALYs at $30,000, the average cost per QALY produced by the two interventions is $10,000 and $6,000 respectively. Intervention A produces five additional QALYs for $70,000 — that is, the incremental cost effectiveness yield is $14,000. In terms of cost effectiveness intervention B is the best.

If a clinician adopts intervention A, he is behaving inefficiently and, in a cash limited health-care system, such behaviour means that potential patients (e.g., in the waiting list) are deprived of care from which they could benefit. Thus, inefficiency is unethical and an ethical practitioner is obliged to demonstrate that he uses society's scarce resources efficiently. The challenge for decisionmakers is to ensure that the institutions of a health-care system create a network of financial and non-financial (e.g., professional rules of conduct) incentives which induce efficient behaviour in providers in particular.

The United Kingdom National Health Service (NHS) is characterized by universal coverage of the population for a comprehensive package of care that is largely "free" (i.e., zero priced) at the point of consumption. It is funded by a global cash limited budget with single-pipe financing (largely from general taxation) and the hospital budget is allocated by means of a weighted capitation formula (the allocation of primary care is demand determined). The recent reforms of the NHS were the product of concern — not about cost containment, but about inefficiency in the use of scarce NHS resources — are epitomized by large variations in clinical practice and the widespread use of interventions of unproven cost effectiveness.

The 1989 reform of the NHS created a purchaser-provider split in which purchasers contract with providers, both public and private. The bulk of NHS "trade" is between near-monopoly local Trust hospitals which trade with and create their income from near-monopsony local purchasers. The introduction of NHS Trust hospitals (which have slightly greater independence but remain publicly owned) and a supplementary system of purchasers based on primary care (general practice fund-holding now covers 40 percent of the population) has been cumulative since 1991.

The government was reluctant to evaluate these reforms (i.e., be "confused" by facts!) and their comprehensive if cumulative introduction has made evaluation difficult because of the absence of controls. The transactions costs of creating and sustaining a market appear to be considerable. The debate about the "success" of the reforms has focused on activity (e.g., completed consultant episodes) and waiting times for non-elective procedures.

Government politicians assert that these reforms have been a "success." It is very difficult to separate out the effects of reform, the effects of recent large cash injections into the NHS, and the cumulative effects of management changes introduced in the mid-1980s. The number of evaluations of Trusts is small and based on the "first wave" (1991-92) group which were atypical. The evaluation of general practice fund-holding (GPFH) is limited: the initial favourable effects on drug prescribing and referrals have disappeared subsequently. Such ignorance of benefit has not prevented the government from deciding to introduce a radical form of GPFH in which fund-holders will hold the total health-care budget for their patients rather than, as at present, just a budget limited to pharmaceuticals, hospital referrals (for diagnostic tests), and a limited range of non-emergency elective surgical procedures.

The conventional wisdom among reformers is that the creation of a market mechanism is the most appropriate way to increase the efficiency of health-care systems. In the United States the advocacy of managed care by Alain Enthoven has produced increasingly more complex proposals to create and sustain market competition (Enthoven 1980; Ellwood et al. 1992). The evidence base for these proposals is slight and relates to early forms of health maintenance organizations that existed in the early 1980s and not to the myriad of for-profit managed care organizations that exist today. These groups are reducing costs in some areas of the United States (e.g., California and New York) but it is not clear whether these savings are genuine (i.e., the product of reducing the volume and price of cost-ineffective care) or the result of aggressive purchasing which has reduced the insurance benefits package and thereby access to cost-effective care.

In Britain, as in the United States, the policy issue is how managed care markets should be regulated. In all sectors of the economy there is regulation. Regulation may be the product of private (e.g., medical associations) and public (e.g., federal or provincial government) action and it will be used to constrain the setting and movement of prices, quality, and volume.

Private sector regulation is typically aimed at enhancing the interests of managing capitalists who, by restricting the working of the competitive market by blocking the entry of new rivals, act to undermine the competitive process. The eighteenth century Scottish political economist Adam Smith argued that "people of the same trade rarely meet together, even for merriment and diversion, but the conversation ends in a conspiracy against the public or in some contrivance to raise prices."

The decision by the Dutch, New Zealand, and British governments to create health-care markets brings with it the issue of how the self-interest of public and private consumers at "the health-care feast" is to be regulated for the public good. A market is a network of buyers and sellers and such networks, whether public or private, are always regulated. The behaviour of providers and purchasers is a product of this regulatory environment.

Who should set the rules for health-care markets? The inference of both Enthoven's advocacy and practice in the United States and Europe is that government must set the "rules of engagement" in health-care markets. Thus, in principle markets decentralize decisionmaking to the local level but in practice government will regulate the market to ensure that its goals of cost control, equity, and efficiency are achieved.

What sort of areas does government have to control? The first area is price setting. The role of the price mechanism is, in principle, to signal to decisionmakers whether there is relative scarcity or abundance in a market. If the harvest is good, prices will fall and may affect future planting (supply) decisions. If the harvest is poor, prices will rise and encourage future planting and supply.

Prices may also reflect monopoly (sole seller) and monopsony (sole buyer). Thus in the UK-NHS reforms, the minister realized that that freedom of price setting might enable near-monopoly local Trusts hospitals to raise prices and corrupt the signalling role of the price mechanism. He therefore set the rule that price should equal average cost.

In a health-care system like the NHS where financial data about costs (as opposed to income and expenditure) is practically absent, price setting is very "approximate." Even if the government had the means to monitor adherence to its costing rule, its logic is poor, being related to financial expediency rather than economic efficiency. In competitive markets prices typically reflect contract terms, for example, a large contract over many years will have a lower unit offer price than a small, short-term contract. To restrict pricing discretion in the way British ministers did, was to act in a way that impaired market efficiency.

Another important regulatory decision concerns the creation and operation of a capital market. If private capital funding is encouraged this reduces pressure on public finance but means that cost-containment policies may be less effective. Typically, in most health-care markets, it is not price competition but "quality competition." This means that, for instance, hospitals compete on ambience (the pile of the carpets!) and the conspicuous consumption of high technology. Such competition may be facilitated by liberal capital market rules and may inflate costs, but has minimal impact on the effectiveness of interventions.

The cost savings apparently produced by managed competition in the US appear to have been produced by radical changes in the skill mix. The evidence base to support the substitution of, for instance, doctors for nurses is dated and limited (Richardson and Maynard 1995) but this has not inhibited US managers who have invested heavily in the primary care gatekeeper (for which there is no evidence but widespread enthusiasm!), nurse practitioners, and care assistants. If Canada takes the health-care market route, will skill mix alterations be at the discretion of managers and subject only to trade union opposition? Will the payment for labour be decided centrally or locally?

The market option often leads to the market testing of services — inviting tenders from competing public and private providers. A list of services that were market tested recently in the UK-NHS is shown in Table 2.

Table 2:   Recent Market Testing in the UK and NHS

• Anaesthetics	• MRI
• Chiropody	• OT
• Clinical genetics	• Pathology
• Continuing care: elderly	• Pharmacy
• Haematology	• Physiotherapy
• Infection control	• Prosthetics
• IZV ophthalmology	• Radiology
• Lithotripsy	• Speech Therapy

Source: Author's compilation.

Whether savings from such policies are "one-off" or continuous and cumulative is disputed.

Markets can be created in many shapes and forms and each one has different regulatory rules and different incentive structures. The available evidence about the efficiency of markets as mechanisms to create system efficiency, equity, and cost containment should not lead any Canadian policymaker to be optimistic that a "miracle cure" for the problems of their health-care system is on hand! Often markets create even worse problems than the ones they were devised to remedy (Hsiao 1994). Unfortunately such evidence rarely curbs the enthusiasm of politicians convinced they have found the Holy Grail of a "solution" to all the ill-defined problems of their health-care system!

CONCLUSIONS

The Canadian, Swedish, German, British, and New Zealand systems perform moderately well. The usual cause of increasing expenditure is the desire of providers to enhance their income and employment: the patient's health, as demonstrated by evidence of the cost effectiveness of new therapies, is not always (rarely?) the concern of those advocating increased expenditure. With existing policies, in particular global budgets, single-pipe financing and disdain for user charges, it is possible to control expenditure provided federal and provincial politicians are not seeking to buy votes through expenditure inflation or privatization "scams" in the run-up to an election.

The primary policy problem in most civilized (non-US) health-care systems is how to enhance the efficiency with which scarce health-care resources are used: the equity and cost-containment problems are quite well controlled. The costs of creating and sustaining competitive market mechanisms to achieve greater efficiency are high and it is necessary, by careful policy evaluation, to demonstrate that these costs are more than compensated for by the efficiency gains created by competition and do not undermine equity and cost-control policies.

Perhaps the most important effect of the market approach is the greater clarity in the specification of contracts, that is, the obligations of providers in terms of delivery to agreed cost, quality, and volume objectives. The purchaser role has been identified and empowered and these managers instead of being price-takers have become often aggressive price-makers. However, efficient price-making can only be done with collaboration between decisionmakers. The health-care reform issue in terms of the induction of efficient behaviour by providers, is what is the optimal combination of competition, collaboration, and cooperation? The latter incentives, the essence of professionalism, should not be discarded carelessly in preference for the uncharted and unproven waters of competition.

The decentralization of decisionmaking using, for instance, market reforms may make the achievement of efficiency, equity, and cost containment more difficult to attain. Perhaps cost inflation, greater inefficiency, and increased inequality are desired by some Canadians — those, such as income maximizing physicians, who prefer the development of private health care insurance to fund private care. In the end policy choices reflect social values as interpreted, however imperfectly, by elected politicians. The academic inevitably hopes that such choices will be informed by evidence and caution. Simple solutions for complex problems rarely exist and should be treated with scepticism. As Mark Twain remarked "whenever you are on the side of the majority, it is time to pause and reflect"!

References

Carr-Hill, R., G. Hardman, S. Peacock, T.A. Sheldon. and P. Smith. 1994. "Allocating Resources to Health Authorities: A Small Area Analysis of Inpatient Utilisation I: Background and Methods." *British Medical Journal* 309:1046-1049.

Ellwood, P.M., A.C. Enthoven, L. Etheridge. 1992. "The Jackson Hole Initiatives for a Twenty-First Century American Health Care System," *Health Economics* 1, 3:169-180.

Enthoven, A.C. 1980. *Health Plan*. Reading, MA: Addison-Wesley.

Grossman, M. 1972. *The Demand for Health*. Chicago: Chicago University Press, National Bureau for Economic Research.

Hsiao, W.C. 1994. "Marketization — The Illusory Magic Pill." *Health Economics* 3, 6:351-357.

Judge, K. 1995. *Tackling Inequalities in Health: An Agenda for Action*. London: Kings Fund.

Maynard, A. 1994. "Can Competition Enhance Efficiency in Health Care? Lessons from the Reform of the UK National Health Service," *Social Science Medicine* 39, 10:1433-1445.

McKeown, J. 1974. *The Modern Rise of Population*. Oxford: Basil Blackwell

Peacock, S. and P. Smith. 1995. *The Resource Allocation Consequences of the New NHS Needs Formula*. Discussion Paper no.134. York: Centre for Health Economics, University of York.

Reinhardt, U. 1978. "Table Manners at the Health Care Feast. In *Financing Health Care: Competition Versus Regulation*, ed. D. Yaggy and W.A. Anylan. Cambridge, MA: Ballinger.

Richardson, G. and A. Maynard. 1995. *Fewer Doctors? More Nurses? A Review of the Knowledge Base of Doctor-Nurse Substitution*. Discussion Paper no. 135. York: Centre for Health Economics, University of York.

Smith, A. 1776, 1976. *An Inquiry into the Nature and Causes of a Wealth of Nations*. Oxford: Oxford University Press.

Smith, P., T.A. Sheldon, R.A. Carr-Hill, G. Hardman, S. Martin and S. Peacock. 1994. "Allocating Resources to Health Authorities: A Small Area Analysis of Inpatient Utilisation II: Results and Policy Implications," *British Medical Journal* 309:1050-1054.

Stoddart, G.L., M.L. Barer and R.D. Evans. 1994. *User Changes, Snares and Delusions: Another Look at the Literature*. Toronto: Premier's Council on Health, Well-Being and Social Justice.

Wennberg, J.E. 1993. "Future Directions for Small Area Variations," *Medical Care* 31:5:Y575-Y580.

Wolfe, P.R. and D.W. Moran. 1993. "Global Budgeting in OECD Countries," *Health Care Financing* 14, 3:55-76.

New Zealand

Malcolm Anderson

INTRODUCTION

The purpose of this paper is to shed some light on the nature and extent of the recent health reforms in New Zealand as they relate to issues of regionalization and decentralization. Given that there is considerable interest in the New Zealand reforms internationally it is hoped that the paper will provide some details that enrich the understanding of what has taken place (*Health Policy* 1994).

The first section of the paper provides the context for understanding the reforms. The second section outlines some of the main problems cited with the pre-reform health-care delivery system and describes the changes that have taken place with the reforms. Section Three focuses on the question of scale — the appropriate level of which is central to any discussion on decentralization and regionalization. Regional variation across the regional health authorities is outlined and specific attention is directed to how planning is addressed by the Southern Regional Health Authority (SRHA), which is responsible for delivering care to the most geographically dispersed population of the four RHAs. Section Four discusses how the reforms are perceived — an important consideration that often determines the success or failure of any reform process. The final section summarises some of the key themes from the New Zealand experience and points to lessons that can be learned for policymakers in Canada.

CONTEXT

New Zealand is a relatively small industrialized country of approximately 3.5 million people. Of that 3.5 million, just over 13 percent are Maori (the indigenous people), and 5 percent are Pacific Islanders mainly from Tonga, Samoa, Niue, Fiji and the Cook Islands. Like other industrial countries the population is aging. In 1994, 11.8 percent of the population was over age 65, compared to 10.2 percent in 1984. The Maori and Pacific Islanders, however, have a much younger profile, similar to those of developing countries, with about twice the number of children aged 15 and under compared to the rest of the New Zealand population.

In geographical terms, the entire country can be placed within the province of Ontario two and a half times, and very few communities are more than two hours drive to the coast. Most of the population is concentrated in the warmer North Island, particularly around Auckland. There has been a continual rural to urban population shift and also an increasing proportion of the population living on the North Island (85 percent of the population is urban).

Since the mid-1980s the country has undergone substantial and rapid social and economic reforms. The underlying current of the reform process has been the move to a more efficient, market-based economy. Government expenditures in health and social services have been contained, the economy has been deregulated and protection for local businesses has been removed. Welfare-based principles, which for so long characterized the country, have been replaced by a culture that, to some observers, is "more American than the United States."

Since the "reforms" began in 1984 both dominant political parties, Labour and National, have sought to turn the economy around. Today, exports have climbed 70 percent in the past three years, economic growth has been about 5 percent over the past few years, and the government runs a surplus. According to a recent *Globe and Mail* article (3 June 1995), NZ's accumulated foreign debt will be paid off by 1998. This growth has been at the expense of declining welfare, increases in violent crime and an unemployment rate that for several years ran at very high levels (it is now down to approximately 7 percent). There have been continual calls, or demands, that Canada learn from NZ's experience, especially since it appears to be in a similar situation to that which New Zealand faced in the mid-1980s. Health-care reform is just one of the areas that deserves closer attention.

Total health expenditure for NZ in 1992-93 was $5.8 billion. Of this, approximately $4.65 billion was publicly financed (i.e., 76.5 percent down from 88 percent in 1979-80). Private expenditure on health care totalled 18 percent (up from 10 percent in 1979-80) while health insurers spent 5.2 percent of the total (up from 1.2 percent in 1979-80).

REFORMS

A Brief History

In the 1950s, hospitals were generally operated as local authorities, each with elected boards with funding derived from local land tax revenues and government subsidies. In 1957 the central government assumed responsibility for funding with the elected boards remaining intact. Funding remained based on the historical pattern, and this continued the uneven access to services across the country. Hospital services were free to the consumer. Primary care was provided by private practitioners with the central government subsidizing only part of the costs of each visit (this proportion declined from about 75 percent in 1941 to an average of between 20-30 percent in 1986). Long-term care was provided by hospitals, with community care provided mainly by volunteer agencies and some private rest homes.

Between 1979 and 1989 total expenditure on health increased from $4.45 billion to $5.49 billion (deflated). Publicly funded services declined from 88 percent of total expenditure in 1979 to 82.6 percent in 1989 (the decline continued to 76.5 percent in 1992). With rising costs throughout the 1980s there were a number of ad hoc reform measures put in place. District offices of the Department of Health, primarily responsible for public health and regulatory services, were integrated with hospital boards into 14 Area Health Boards (AHBs). The AHBs were funded through global budgets based, in part, on population-based funding formulas. AHBs had a fair degree of discretion over how the funds were spent. AHBs were responsible for hospital-based services and public health, although the Department of Health continued to run national health promotion campaigns. Essentially the AHBs acted as both purchasers and providers.

A number of reviews in the late 1980s concluded that the health-care system was in need of radical reform. The 1987 Gibbs report recommended a provider-purchaser split in which public hospitals would become independent, competing businesses and district health authorities (precursors to AHBs) would contract with providers for services. Although similar proposals were being proposed in the UK the New Zealand government decided to continue with slower, incremental change. Contracts were introduced between the central government and the AHBs, and the locally elected boards were now enhanced by appointed members. The government also introduced ad hoc measures aimed at curbing increasing costs. These measures included user charges for Rx drugs and renewed emphasis on generic drugs, limiting subsidies for GP visits, an attempt to switch GPs from FFS to contracts, and the removal of annual price and wage adjustments for AHBs.

PROBLEMS WITH THE PRE-REFORM SYSTEM

The newly elected National party government in 1990 put a renewed emphasis on health-care reform. In the government's 1991 document "Your Health and Public Health" several key problems with the existing system were identified. The report recommended a number of substantial reforms that were influenced by changes occurring in the Netherlands and the UK. These problems included:

Waiting Times

Waiting times, the report claimed, were too long and in some places poorly managed — with many people having to wait for public hospital surgery for more than a year. In some places, for example, "urgent" hip replacements had a one- to three-year waiting time, while the "routine" hip replacements wait was between two and four years. AHBs, it was argued, were responding to funding constraints by decreasing services — especially since there were no incentives to look at more innovative and efficient ways to deliver services. For ENT in one large AHB, it was noted that 15 percent of the waiting list no longer required surgery and the eligibility of others was questioned since they just wanted to have their noses straightened (appropriateness). In addition, there was considerable anecdotal evidence to suggest that private consultations received quicker services in public facilities than public consulting patients, and that the pressures were exacerbated by using acute care beds when rehabilitative care would have been more appropriate.

Area Health Boards

AHBs both purchased and provided services. This perceived conflicting role suggested to many that AHBs were using their own facilities, however less cost-effective and less appropriate when compared to other suppliers, as this would minimize staff losses and undercapacity facilities (questions here of demand versus need). There was little incentive, the report claimed, for AHBs to move to community, day-stay or out-patient care.

There was also imprecise role definition among the AHBs, government, and communities. Elected board members were responsible to the communities that appointed them, but then were not responsible for raising the money the boards allocated (governance issues).

Many other issues were cited as problematic. These included poor management skills, limited use of clinical databases and cost analyses, lack of appropriate systems for evaluating the quality of care, and poor systems for funding continuing care for the "physically, intellectually and psychology disabled and the frail elderly."

Fragmented Funding

A major problem cited was the fragmentation of funding with different parts of the system funded in different ways (inappropriate use of financial resources). Funding to AHBs was based on an adjusted population basis, primary care was provided through a mix of subsidies, some accident related services were paid for through the Accident Compensation Corporation, and the funding of physically, intellectually and psychology disabled, and the frail elderly was arbitrary and inconsistent among the AHBs. Moreover, the funding fragmentation contributed to the poor management, allocation, and integration of appropriate, patient-specific care. Cost-shifting also occurred as some health professionals diverted patients to services that would be provided faster even though they were less appropriate.

Accessibility to Services

Anecdotal evidence suggests that access to care is compounded by user-charges for GP consultations and prescription drug costs. People on low incomes were reluctant to use the services sooner — which resulted in worsening health status and then eventual admission into the system at a greater cost (e.g., hospital admission). Despite the small size of New Zealand, geographical access to care was seen as uneven across the country with obvious rural-urban differences and some locations being particularly overserviced (e.g., Dunedin in the South Island). Furthermore, appropriate services tailored to the needs of different ethnic groups were strongly recommended and desired and the existing structure was not considered capable of delivering this effectively.

Lack of Consumer Control

Several submissions to review boards on health care indicated that consumers and communities (geographical, cultural, and illness-specific "communities") were not adequately engaged in the process of resource allocation and need identification. Given that people are perceived to want a greater say in how their health care is delivered, the existing structure did not enhance the different communities' ability to do so.

Fairness

As a backdrop to many of these issues, there were inconsistencies in the funding allocation mechanism, subsidies for services, and the criteria for private and public hospital treatment. The structure could not adequately respond to location and culture specific needs for different types of care and this contributed to the inequality of access across the country.

Based on the overriding pressures of fiscal restraint and the above concerns, it was strongly recommended that a substantial overhaul of the health-care system was required. Given the context — one in which New Zealanders were facing considerable reengineering in a number of other social, economic, and political dimensions, it was not surprising that health care was targeted for so-called "reform."

REFORMS AND THE NEW ORGANIZATIONAL STRUCTURE

The New Zealand government introduced a number of fundamental reforms in July 1993 — the basis of which was the policy green and white paper, *Your Health and Public Health*, released in 1991. The reforms included the following:

- integrated funding (for personal health, community services, primary, secondary and tertiary care);
- separation of purchaser and provider roles;
- explicit statement of the "core health services" to be publicly funded;
- separation of public and personal health services;
- competition among providers.

Missing from the initial reform package promoted in 1991 was explicit reference to competition between purchasers, a plan to apply social insurance to fund health care, and the use of part-charges for in-patient care and a softening of the definition and role of core services. In essence, the initial proposals were subjected to, and transformed by, the political and implementation realities of the health-care environment.

The new structure put in place with these reforms is shown in Figure 1. The AHBs, which were both providers and purchasers of personal (mainly secondary care) and public health services were replaced by:

- four Regional Health Authorities (RHAs) which now purchase all personal health and disability services;
- 23 Crown Health Enterprises (CHEs) the new publicly-owned providers, which are based on the major public hospitals across the country;
- a Public Health Commission, which purchased public health services aimed at populations (which, as of July 1995, has been dismantled);
- a National Advisory Committee on Core Health and Disability Support Services (Core Services Committee);
- a distinct monitoring agency to oversee the functioning of the CHEs; and
- a new Ministry of Health, which develops policy, negotiates and monitors the purchasers and administers public health regulations.

Figure 1: Organization of the Health Sector, 1993

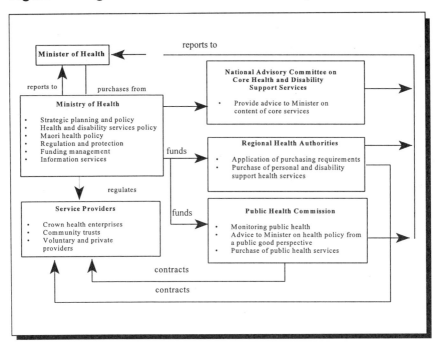

Source: *Your Health and Public Health*, NZ Ministry of Health.

While the overall goal of the reforms has been debated, the government in particular has been optimistic that the new structures will eventually enhance efficiencies, provide innovative, more appropriate and higher quality care, and will be far more cost effective compared to the previous structure.

Funding

Over 90 percent of the $4.65 billion spent on publicly-funded health care in 1993-94 went to the RHAs. Funding is determined by an equitable population-based formula, although it is anticipated that equity among the RHAs will not be fully achieved for a few years.

There are four broad elements of the purchasing cycle: policy, funding negotiation, purchasing, and monitoring. Each year the government issues *policy guidelines* which show its strategic direction for health care over the short term and any priorities it wishes to focus on (normally in the November prior to the purchase year). The RHAs (purchasers) must then develop purchase plans in response to the guidelines and develop a *funding agreement* with the minister of health by July 1st (the beginning of the financial year). These plans must include the direction the RHA is taking in each of the four priority areas (i.e., Maori health, child health, mental health, and health of the physical environment). The *purchasing of services* continues throughout the year. The purchasers *monitor* the providers to ensure the level and quality of care is being provided. The RHAs report on a quarterly basis to the ministry so the ministry can determine if the purchasers are meeting their funding commitment. Finally, the RHAs are required to made a public report (an annual report) regarding their performance about three months from the year end.

Roles and Responsibilities of RHAs

The fundamental cornerstone of the NZ reforms is the purchaser-provider split through the formation of RHAs. Early analyses conducted by the NZ government suggested that the appropriate number of RHAs required for effective and efficient services was between three and six. Based on reviewing a number of issues such as the optimal number for funding allocation, contracting, monitoring, and community representation, it was decided that four would be the optimal number — that is, ultimately it was a political decision! (A profile of each RHA is provided in Table 1.)

Each RHA is required to purchase health and disability services for its region, determine the needs for these services, monitor the performance of purchasing relationships with providers and engage in a consultative process with individuals and organizations in the communities it serves. The RHAs do not provide any health service, but rather plan and purchase these services. In the first year of the reforms the RHAs were required to "rollover" existing relationships, or purchase the same level and range of services as prior to the reforms. The range and level is being reviewed by the Core Services Committee.

RHA Boards are appointed by the minister of health, with whom the RHA has a contract to purchase a range of services for the region. As well as purchasing secondary and tertiary hospital services, community and disability support services, and environmental/public health services that were

Table 1: Breakdown of Funding and Population by RHA, 1993-1994 ($million)

Region	Personal Health	Disability Support	Total	Population*
Northern	1,012.28	327.10	1,339.38	1,133,300
Midland	664.48	198.12	862.60	703,900
Central	814.21	286.16	1,100.37	874,000
Southern	743.33	252.98	996.31	756,000
New Zealand	3,234.30	1,064.36	4,298.66	3,467,200

*Note: Based on 1993 population projections. In 1993-94, Northern and Midland were underfunded and Central and Southern were overfunded. The government intends to move all RHAs to equity over the next few years.

previously funded by AHBs, the RHAs are responsible for purchasing all primary care such as GPs, pharmaceuticals, and diagnostic services. These services are paid for through public funding and private payment by individuals.

Contracting, Administration, and Monitoring

One of the key strengths perceived early in the reform process was the ability to provide better services through competition. Contracting has numerous advantages. These include: increased opportunities for innovation, contracts that fit the specific needs of communities (geographic, population, and illness-specific), and, from the government's perspective, when determined regionally or subregionally, contracts minimize the opportunity for nationally-based organizations to skew the government's planning intentions. The government has made reference to the fact that negotiations with the NZ Medical Association have often been difficult, but with the evolutionary move towards regionally-based relationships the power-base of the national organization will be eroded.

One of the major criticisms of contracting, however, is the cost incurred. Each of the four RHAs, for example, has its own approach to contracting

— which to some observers, results in the duplication of costs. The government maintains that the relatively high costs encountered are related to the current period of transition and the high start-up costs of developing the contractual relationships with providers (e.g., determining the contracting environment, contract structure, the degree of detail required for service specification). There are only a small number of contracts with providers at the national level (see Table 2) so a reduction in the number of RHAs would not necessarily reduce the extent of contracting. Table 2 also reflects the variation, just in costs of contracting alone, among the RHAs. Each RHA has a different approach to contracting secondary and tertiary services. In the northern and midland regions the RHAs and CHEs work downwards from an aggregate price level and determine the individual service prices from that amount. In contrast, central and southern RHAs work upwards from specific contract prices for services, which are then added up to a total price paid.

The government anticipates considerable savings in primary care and community-based services through budget-holding and capitation contracts. For fundholders, there is the opportunity for benefit-sharing while at the same time there are no risks incurred. An RHA may contract a group of physicians or a community trust, for example, to provide a range of services

Table 2: Estimated Costs of Contracting, 1994

Contracting Costs	Northern	Midland	Central	Southern
CHEs (exc.GST)	$1,250,000	$1,200,000	$650,000	$473,700 (8 months)
IHC (Intellectually Handicapped)	$ 9,500	$ 9,000	$ 10,000	$ 7,897
Plunket	$ 3,500	$ 3,742	$ 11,000	$ 3,256
Rest Homes	not yet negotiated	$ 37,917	$ 70,000	$ 24,540

Source: Memorandum for the Cabinet Committee on Social Assistance Reforms, Office of the Minister of Health, NZ Government.

for a given population group. If the fundholder provides the required care within the budget and has a "surplus," it is allowed to retain the savings and invest in new equipment, facilities, programs and so on to further improve the nature of care it provides. If the fundholder exceeds the notional budget, then that loss is absorbed by the RHA. The Pegasus fundholding group of GPs in Christchurch, for example, has already reduced laboratory costs by 30 percent. There are a number of fundholders now emerging across the country which contract with both the RHAs and the CHEs. RHAs predict that over half the GPs will be in some form of fundholding or managed care relationship by the end of the 1995-96 fiscal year (Lovelace 1995).

The government estimates that while there would be a reduction in administrative costs with fewer RHAs, these gains would be offset by the need to establish more district offices and travel times to subregions around the country, and the fact that RHAs would still have to contract with the same number of subregional providers. Again, much of the concern regarding these costs, contends the government, is based on the high start-up costs incurred in this period of transition. Already, however, it is noticeable that some RHAs have been more effective than others in the administration costs. For the 1994-95 fiscal year, northern RHA's budgeted costs for administration came to $13.20 per capita, while midland's costs ran to $17.87 per capita (central RHAs administration costs were $14.67 per capita and southern's $17.50).

The ministry of health undertake monitoring and reviews of the RHAs to ensure that appropriate services are being planned and purchased. The ministry also intends to review the roles and responsibilities of the RHA boards, strategic visions, risk management, organizational size, function and operating budgets, and the organizational culture. The ministry will also monitor the overhead and administrative costs of the RHAs.

Although the new structure has only been in place for a short period of time, the RHAs have begun to work together on some purchasing strategies. In addition to sharing their collective information and experiences they have worked together on purchasing strategies for pharmaceuticals and some tertiary services. As the process of reform continues it is expected that the RHAs will continuously improve the way they operate as they learn from one another.

Crown Health Enterprises (CHEs)

CHEs negotiate contracts with RHAs to provide hospital and related services. In order for a CHE to get a contract with an RHA the CHE must provide those services at a price and quality that is acceptable to the RHA. They were also contracted with the Public Health Commission prior to its disestablishment. CHEs function under the framework of commercial law (*Companies Act* and the *Commerce Act*), and are required to implement policy which prevents their resources being used for "private" consumers at the expense of RHA-funded individuals.

CHEs have been under considerable pressure in their new role. They have inherited substantial debt from their earlier incarnations, to the extent that commercial banks were not willing to offer loans to the new enterprises. The government has sought to redress the issue by providing the RHAs with additional funding that will allow the CHEs to recover their costs and restructure their debt-equity ratios.

Within the CHEs there have been some noticeable organizational changes. At South Auckland Health CHE, for example, following an organizational review it was found that there were more managers than required and subsequently many managers were made redundant. The money freed up was used to employ more clinical staff to improve the service provided. Staff are now regularly surveyed about job satisfaction and there has been a cultural shift with a greater focus being placed on the customer. Moreover, the CHE is improving communications with other providers and voluntary community groups in the area to improve customer-focused service provision. Another CEO in the South Island has commented that

> it would be fair to say that the clinical staff I work with have greeted the health reforms with a degree of cynicism in terms of "yet another management change." I believe that they have subsequently turned around to some extent to now wish to work with management to achieve some goals. The significant reason for the turnaround is the recognition by management that unless they are working with clinicians no gains are going to be achieved. (Personal communication).

Accountability is another feature of the NZ reforms, which, to many health-care workers has been long overdue. As one CHE chairperson commented with regard to the perceived "americanization" of the NZ health system:

to develop hospitals according to basic business principles ensures that there will be someone who is responsible and can account for the expenditure of public money in health. Previously, under the old health system, there was no such accountability and there was no justification for a lot of money spent on buying equipment or building new hospitals. (Personal communication)

The reform process has created both a necessity and an opportunity for organizational change in CHEs. Clearly, the combination of accountability, effective management, improved integration between management and clinicians, and the increasing use of management and case mix information systems should contribute to improving the quality of care in a cost-effective manner.

Core Services Committee

The primary function of the Core Services Committee (CSC) was to assess the effectiveness and priority of health and disability support services and to advise which services should be publicly funded. To some observers, the central criticism of the committee has been that it has not attempted to define a comprehensive list of core services (the Ministry of Health has instead begun to develop a list of core services so that the minimum standards of access can be established). The CSC has, however, played a leading role in recommending the terms of access to certain services (e.g., ambulance, overseas medical coverage and dental treatment for low-income adults), and has been instrumental in developing best-practice guidelines for diagnosing and managing specific conditions.

SCALE

A central feature of the reform package, in place now for almost two years, has been the devolution of decisionmaking to the RHAs, which, in turn, contract for services to the providers within their respective areas, and with other RHAs. There is then, an explicit geographical dimension to the new structure. But does this provide equity of care throughout the country and how is planning conducted at the RHA level?

One of the underlying themes has been to develop a more efficient system that provides equal access to services that are responsive to the needs of the location and culture-specific communities. This will take time. As examiners of the new system as a whole, it becomes a question of the most appropriate scale for providing integrated, needs-specific care evenly across the country.

Regional Variation

If we look at the country as a whole, cross-regional comparisons of RHAs show variation in a number of different measures. As Tables 1 to 5 suggest, we can see this variation with regard to funding allocation, contracting costs, average length of stay and daycase surgery discharges. These broader figures, however, although alluding to distinct variation at the regional scale, mask the differences that are also apparent at the intraregional scale. It is at this point where appropriate planning is critical to the fulfilment of optimal equity-based service provision across the country. The following section focuses on the case of the Southern Regional Health Authority (SRHA) to illustrate the existence of disparities at the intra-RHA level and to provide a concrete example of how planning at this scale is conducted.

More importantly, the SRHA is used as a case study of the planning approach the NZ government has recommended to all RHAs — namely the adoption of a distance and time-based planning strategy for access to services. The time-distance approach has been regarded as a "pioneering step" in regionalized health-care delivery. The determination of "appropriate" times for accessing services was based on current levels of access, geography, and the professional judgement of chief advisors in the Ministry of Health. The RHAs were also consulted on the approach.

Southern Regional Health Authority (SRHA)

In New Zealand it has been the SRHA that has lead the way in the development of this approach since the early 1990s. The pressure for such a planning strategy was motivated by the region's awareness that it would have to rationalize its services in the reformed system because historically it was overfunded.

Table 3: Expenditure per Head of Population for the RHAs, 1994

Regional Health Authority	Expenditure Per Head
Northern	$1,049
Midland	$1,079
Central	$1,106
Southern	$1,152

Note: Funding for many years was based on historical levels despite a faster population growth rate in the North Island.
Source: *Purchasing for Your Health*, NZ Ministry of Health.

Table 4: Average Length of Stay in CHEs*

Operations by CHEs	Northern RHA	Midland RHA	Central RHA	Southern RHA
Angioplasty	6.2	4.7	4.2	6.2
Carpal tunnel release	1.1	0.4	0.4	0.4
Cataract	1.7	1.5	1.7	1.3
Coronary artery bypass	14.8	13.4	15.7	15.7
Hip replacement	14.7	15.5	13.9	14.4
Hysterectomy	6.0	6.1	6.2	6.3
Knee replacement	13.4	13.8	12.7	12.1
Prostatectomy	6.3	5.6	6.1	7.3
Repair of hernia	2.7	2.0	2.4	2.5

Note: *12 months to June 1994.
Source: *Purchasing for Your Health*, NZ Ministry of Health.

Table 5: Percent of Daycase Surgery Discharges by CHEs*

Daycase Discharges by CHEs	Northern RHA	Midland RHA	Central RHA	Southern RHA
Blood, immunity	18.3	28.5	48.4	31.9
Burns	1.4	7.4	5.9	3.7
Cancer	14.2	20.3	17.3	13.5
Circulatory system	4.3	11.7	6.1	14.4
Digestive system	8.8	20.7	21.2	21.0
ENT and mouth	56.4	52.9	45.3	51.9
Endocrine, nutrition	2.8	5.0	5.0	7.3
Eye	20.2	32.4	22.8	42.6
Infections, parasites	5.7	8.6	11.7	11.6
Injury	6.7	10.4	15.8	12.1
Kidney, urinary tract	17.3	15.6	15.3	16.0
Liver, pancreas	1.6	7.1	10.6	7.7
Muscoskeletal system	9.4	15.6	20.9	15.4
Nervous system	26.6	38.4	40.1	39.1
Pregnancy, birth	3.1	4.1	3.9	4.7
Respiratory system	3.3	32.3	11.9	8.4
Female reproductive system	47.0	49.2	51.1	49.6
Male reproductive system	12.2	22.7	21.9	22.4
Total discharges by CHE	25.2	29.2	28.9	30.1

Note: *12 months to June 1994. Casemix adjusted day cases.
Source: *Purchasing for Your Health*, NZ Ministry of Health.

Although it is the largest RHA geographically, covering almost half of the country and most of the South Island the SRHA purchases services for just 23 percent of New Zealand's population (approximately 740,000 people). Tertiary services are based on the more populated east coast in Christchurch (300,000 people) and Dunedin (120,000), where there is a medical school. Several other hospitals are located in smaller towns dispersed over the South Island. Many areas within the SRHA have a huge influx of tourists and holiday-makers in the summer (e.g., Central Otago and Fiordland). Although regarded as historically overfunded when compared to the other RHAs, the SRHA contains some of the most isolated communities and it is here and in the smaller towns, where pressures to rationalize have been felt the most. There are five major challenges facing the SRHA (Southern Regional Health Authority 1994):

- geographic — many communities are remote;
- ageing — a steady increase in the number of people aged 60 and over is expected during the next 40 years;
- population-based funding — the region has been overserviced (i.e., more money per capita than the rest of the country) hence pressures to rationalize;
- rising costs of primary care — increasing primary care costs are placing pressures on other services such as hospital-based care;
- current levels of inequitable access to services in the SRHA.

Intra-RHA variation

Within the SRHA there are noticeable variations in services and utilization. As Tables 6 to 8 suggest, the access and nature of care varies from place-to-place, with some of the smaller communities with considerably less "access" to a full range of services compared to the larger centres. This, however, is one of the realities of health-care provision spatially and financially, it is not feasible that all services can be provided to all communities.

The *explicit recognition of limited funding* must be incorporated into planning which is based upon *implicit spatial realities of distance decay*.

Table 6: Percent of Daycase Surgery Discharges by CHEs within the Southern RHA*

Daycase Discharges	Southern RHA	Coast Health Care	Canterbury Health	Healthlink South	Health South Canterbury	Healthcare Otago	Southern Health
Blood, immunity	32.9	80.4	30.2	0.0	34.5	26.8	26.8
Burns	3.7	0.0	7.7	0.0	0.0	0.0	0.0
Cancer	13.5	32.3	14.2	10.4	11.3	11.0	18.1
Circulatory system	14.4	4.1	25.0	0.0	1.6	9.2	13.3
Digestive system	21.0	27.4	24.5	18.4	15.7	16.4	19.3
ENT and mouth	51.9	34.3	49.1	0.0	36.4	60.6	47.8
Endocrine, nutrition	7.5	9.9	9.1	0.0	0.0	7.2	4.1
Eye	42.6	35.2	54.4	181.7	37.1	38.1	21.2
Infections, parasites	11.6	25.0	13.0	0.0	10.0	9.3	12.5
Injury, poisoning	12.1	19.6	9.7	9.7	27.0	10.4	15.5
Kidney, urinary tract	16.0	11.8	15.6	0.0	14.9	20.8	6.6
Liver, pancreas	7.7	0.0	2.0	0.0	9.0	13.8	1.1
Muscoskeletal system	15.4	7.4	19.2	0.0	19.0	13.7	9.5
Nervous system	39.1	42.6	38.6	62.1	36.1	40.3	31.3
Pregnancy, birth	4.7	0.0	0.0	5.7	4.1	3.3	2.1
Respiratory system	8.4	73.7	21.5	0.0	0.0	1.6	13.0
Female reproductive system	49.6	32.6	44.0	52.5	37.7	66.4	35.5
Male reproductive system	22.4	14.1	23.5	27.1	17.0	23.8	20.4
Total discharges by CHE	30.1	27.8	32.5	30.6	25.9	32.3	22.9

Note: *12 months to June, 1994. Casemix adjusted day cases
Source: *Purchasing for Your Health*, NZ Ministry of Health.

Table 7: Average Length of Stay (Days) in the Southern RHA, 1989-1994*

CHE	1989/90	1990/91	1991/92	1992/93	1993/94
Coast Healthcare	7.0	7.5	7.1	5.9	5.4
Health South Canterbury	9.2	9.5	9.9	6.7	6.8
Healthcare Otago	7.8	7.4	7.5	7.0	6.8
Southern Health	7.9	7.5	6.3	6.1	5.4

Note: *Canterbury Health and Healthlink South are excluded due to difficulty in obtaining ALOS data prior to 1993/94.
Source: *Purchasing for Your Health*, NZ Ministry of Health.

Table 8: Daypatient Discharges, 1989-1994 for the Southern RHA*

CHE	1989/90	1990/91	1991/92	1992/93	1993/94	Percent Change 89/90-93/94
Coast Healthcare	930	1,031	1,201	1,361	1,522	63.7
Canterbury	7,203	7,171	10,063	10,979	11,982	66.3
Health South Canterbury	215	298	2,107	2,358	2,729	1,169.3
Healthcare Otago	4,514	5,747	6,148	6,605	6,870	52.2
Southern Health	1,512	1,612	2,611	2,963	2,999	98.3

Note: *Canterbury represents consolidation of data due to difficulties separating Canterbury Health and Healthlink when in earlier Canterbury Area Health Board period.
Source: *Purchasing for Your Health*, NZ Ministry of Health.

The hierarchical ordering of services and facilities is based on these realities and the population base of respective communities. Inevitably, this logic will lead to the rationalization of services that historically have been available in a number of communities. The reform process, induced by the new fiscal realities, has magnified the uneven historical profile of service provision across the SRHA. As a consequence, the planned redistribution of services and facilities is facing considerable opposition by the general public and some health professionals in those communities where the level of care is being reduced.

Hierarchical Planning

A central objective for the SRHA has been to "even-out access" to health and disability services, in a geographical context, over the 1994-97 planning period. To do this, the Authority has taken into account a number of key influences which affect the delivery of care. These include:

- the trend towards community-based care;
- emerging high technology care (e.g., laser therapy);
- continuing "subspecializations" in medicine;
- increasing use of day surgery;
- pharmaceutical use replacing in-patient care;
- increased emphasis on conforming to standards of quality;
- increased use of information technology;
- fiscal restraints; and
- the changing role of ambulance and helicopter.

The interplay of these factors has contributed to both decentralization and centralization tendencies in the provision of health services.

Before proceeding with the proposals, the SRHA undertook two consultative initiatives to engage the community in the planning process. In December 1993, the Authority released a document entitled "Access to Care," to which they received 745 submissions. The focus of the document was planning access to services based on travel times. General support existed for primary care access times, although there were many requests for family planning and STD services to be more accessible than what was proposed. Other services were discussed with access times ranging from 30 minutes to 90 minutes. Not surprisingly, the retention of existing smaller hospitals was strongly supported. The second initiative was a survey conducted in August 1993 of over 5,000 residents selected at random across the SRHA. Again, the focus was distance and times to services, and the survey responses indicated the willingness of the public to access different services at different times.

The results of the initiatives were integrated into the planning framework, which is based on travel time (by motor vehicle), population size, and what is referred to as "locality planning." Locality planning alludes to the recognition that communities vary in terms of age profile, cultural differences, geographical isolation, seasonal variation in population size, and so on. Locality planning, therefore, is designed to incorporate location-specific features to make the service provision more focused on the needs of the community served.

There are four levels of care which correspond to different population sizes. At level A (populations between 2,000 and 10,000), the communities should have access to a basic range of services within 30 minutes travel time. These communities should also have a basic range of in-patient hospital services available to them if they are more than one hour away from their nearest neighbouring community (examples include Queenstown, Te Anau, Akaroa, and Reefton).

Level B services are provided for districts whose catchment areas cover up to 25,000 people. There should be a range of basic hospital services available, but specialist services would be located at a different level in the hierarchy. In-patient care would be carried out by GPs for routine care and uncomplicated pregnancies. Examples of these districts include Ashburton, Oamaru, and the Eastern Southland district. For some areas that have populations of just over 10,000 (e.g., Buller and Kaikoura), the relative geographical isolation is taken into account with the addition of some services normally based in larger communities being considered.

At Level C, the third level of hospital services are provided. These "base" hospitals serve populations of up to 100,000 and should be accessible within 90 minutes for 90 percent of the population. These are the main provincial centres — Invercargill, Timaru, and Greymouth. Hospitals provide a range of in-patient medical and surgical services, radiology and laboratory support, and an expanded range of services for the mentally ill and addiction sufferers when compared to Level B hospitals. Finally, Level D hospital services are provided in cities whose catchment areas are between 250,000 and 500,000—that is, Dunedin and Christchurch (located approximately five hours driving time apart). A full range of tertiary services are available from CHEs based in these cities, although lower volume services are normally located at just one of the centres.

At the northern tip of the SRHA (top of the South Island), the authority purchases services from CHEs based in the Central RHA. All elective work, for example, is contracted to Nelson's CHE. At the moment this is based on historical trends, but as the reform process continues, more assessments will be made as to whether services should be provided "in-house" or contracted out.

Issues

SRHA's approach to planning health services has been regarded as more effective by planners compared to other RHAs because it has sought to fully engage the communities in an open consultation process. Other RHAs, it was noted by some observers, have operated in a much more closed, "backroom" approach, whereby the planning policies decided upon have much less community input. For a population of about 740,000, the SRHA has established 22 district health committees, four women's health advisory groups, five disability support services advisory groups and five Maori health groups. There are also four ethics committees in the region designed to safeguard consumer rights and the rights of participants in research. Despite this structure there is continual pressure placed on the SRHA to become more visible in the community. At the same time, additional pressure is placed on the Authority by the media which is quick to point to potential rationalizations, waiting lists and times and concerns being expressed by health-care providers. The reformed are blamed for much of what is still wrong with the system but there is seldom discussion of the alternatives had the reforms not been put in place.

The 1994-95 funding agreement with the ministry requires that all people in the region have "fair and reasonable access to services." One of the government's objectives is for the RHAs to move towards national intervention rates. To date, the SRHA have identified intervention rates for its five subregions (Canterbury, Otago, West Coast, Southland, and South

Canterbury) and has found variation in the actual and expected rates (based on national levels) of public hospital discharges. The next step is to determine why the variation exists. Other RHAs are looking at similar issues.

The SRHA is facing difficult decisions as it seeks to optimize the location of services across its region. In several of the Level B and Level C locations — for example, Balclutha, Timaru, Oamaru and Ashburton, services are in the process of being withdrawn (in some of these hospitals the annual average occupancy rate has been between 45 and 65 percent). Despite being regarded as overserviced by health planners, this has been met with considerable opposition by these centres, which view the rationalization process as a further attack on rural health. And from a broader socio-economic perspective, it is easier to market a town to prospective new businesses or residents if a wider range of health services can be provided within the community. The SRHA, however, will continue to rationalize services to improve equity and the cost effectiveness of health care within the region. Unlike the other RHAs it has had to make these decisions recognizing that historically many parts of its region were overserviced.

PERCEPTION

The reforms in New Zealand are so recent that there is still considerable uncertainty as to the extent of their success or failure. Internationally there is considerable interest — in part, because they were not incrementally put in place but rather represented a wholesale shift in the structure of health-care delivery. Other industrial countries are also facing hard decisions on restructuring health care and look to the New Zealand experience with the hope of finding something to support or refute new policy objectives.

Within New Zealand there are mixed feelings regarding the reforms. Several physicians have openly criticized the pace and nature of the changes, especially as they face growing waiting lists for some surgical procedures. The government meanwhile, has mounted a substantial promotional campaign and there have been several publications prepared at the national level which document the state of health care and the performance of the system (in particular, data on the performance of RHAs and CHEs). There is still uncertainty and some suspicion at the management level about the roles and interaction between RHAs and the CHEs. GPs, such as those in the Pegasus group, are now looking at more innovative organizational approaches in which to provide care.

It is the general public, however, who are perhaps the most confused of all players in the reform process. The reforms were marketed to New Zealanders as a way for "consumers" to have a greater say in the delivery of health care, and for services to be provided more efficiently. To date, the public has not seen as much as was promised. As one CEO of a CHE commented

> I believe the reforms have also raised the expectations of consumers and were marketed to the market as improving consumer knowledge and choice in service provision.... the public are starting to demand this improvement but that is unlikely to be achieved until the reforms have been "bedded down" over the next two to three years. (Personal communication).

The "average New Zealander" is not that aware of all the changes that have taken place. Apart from name changes, the most visible component of the health-care system — the hospital — appears relatively unchanged for the bulk of the population. But the public does hear through the media stories regarding waiting lists and hospital closures in rural areas. And in parts of the country, such as on the west coast of the South Island, the RHA is relatively unknown, since its offices are on the east coast in Christchurch and Dunedin. There have also been particularly scathing newspaper articles that highlight the consulting costs that CHEs have run up on communications of their new structures, and damaging reports of specialists threatening and actually resigning over the deterioration of care that the reforms have produced.

To many health professionals and administrators, however, the reforms have brought about an opportunity for change and improvement in the system. Greater efficiencies have occurred in many places, and the rationalizations have been regarded by many as long overdue. Despite the immediate uncertainty it is anticipated by many analysts and professionals working in the system that over time the new organizational structures can put in place more cost-effective, integrated, community-based care that responds to the needs of the people being served. There is still considerable work required to educate the public and to cement the new relationships between the ministry, RHAs, CHEs, and practitioners. But as the pace of change slows and opportunities for reflection and long-term planning emerge, it is hoped that the new health-care system will improve the health status of all New Zealanders.

SUMMARY

After two years of substantial and rapid upheaval, the evolving health-care system is reaching a stage whereby the nature and extent of change must subside if positive change is to be made. For many questions about the system, the answer is, as one policymaker observed, "don't know, don't know, don't know"! There is still considerable debate as to whether the reforms have been successful or not, and this divergence is likely to continue for some time.

There are some encouraging signs. Fundholding arrangements appear to be increasing in numbers and scope, specific health initiatives for Maori health are slowly developing, RHAs and CHEs and other providers are beginning to develop improved contracting relationships, transactions costs should decrease, and improved, integrated organizational structures in CHEs are being developed. On the other hand, some observers consider the pace of change too rapid and thus creating heightened uncertainty for many health professionals and other workers in the system. The media is very quick to highlight the worst elements of the reforms, such as personal and financial hardship for people who are victims of long waiting times for care. The population is becoming increasingly concerned that the reforms are not working, but this, in part, is fuelled by the media perception and lack of knowledge concerning the structural reforms that have been implemented.

There appears to be consensus, however, from a variety of different sources, that after two years of reforms, the pace and nature of change should now be minimal. There needs to be time to evaluate fully what has happened and this "down time" in change should provide opportunities for further positive, incremental innovation.

As Salmond, Laugesen and Nelson (1995) recently commented, some fundamental questions must be addressed, and "rapid revolutionary change" does not necessarily create an environment in which they can be addressed.

Their key questions, applicable also in the Canadian context, include: "What values do New Zealanders want embedded in [their] health services, or more generally, what sort of society do [they] want? Do [New Zealanders] see health as an individual responsibility, first and foremost, or do [they] see it more as a collective or civic responsibility?"

One of the understated benefits of the reforms has been the shift in focus to the needs of the population at the local level. This "need" will vary from place to place. The logic of the RHA role is that it will determine those needs and purchase the required services far more appropriately than any other structure. The hierarchical, locality-based planning of the SRHA, which has been promoted by the government as an important tool for other RHAs, attempts to provide care at the appropriate geographical scale. Essentially, that is what regionalization in health care is all about — namely appropriate care at the appropriate geographic scale. Regionally focused care is made all the more important in times of harsh financial realities and fiscal responsibility.

The status and interpretation of New Zealand's health-care reforms vary according to whom you are speaking. For the most part this paper has provided an overview of the reforms that have ensued in the past couple of years. But to many observers within New Zealand there has been considerable concern expressed about the reforms; the motivations for change, scepticism regarding those "public relations" elements that were identified as problems in the previous "system that required attention, the broader political dimension behind the reforms, and the roles played by different consultancy groups in the determination of the reform structure. There is an organization, Coalition for Public Health, based in Wellington but with membership across the country, that provides a counterbalance to the claims and interpretations voiced by the government, RHAs, and the CHEs.

As a backdrop to these issues has been the suspicion that the reforms are an attempt to reduce or remove "risk" from public health "tax dollars," and place this risk onto New Zealanders. In short, moving towards a complete free market/user pay system. The reforms thus far, it is argued, are just the beginning of that transformation. When taken within the context of all the other fundamental changes affecting the country the characterization of a free-market ideology in health care deserves closer attention.

Whether the cup is half-full or half-empty, the common theme is that another round of radical adjustment will prove devastating. It is now time for refocusing and acceptance that not all the changes were positive. It is critical that a level of stability is introduced, that RHAs be given time to establish themselves both administratively and in the eyes of the NZ public, that politics take a back seat, that time be given to fully examine the nature of continuing and new problems that exist after two years of reforms, and that the implementation of future changes be incremental and not "radical" in order to minimize the degree of uncertainty for the purchasers, providers, and the public.

LESSONS LEARNED?

There are several lessons that can be learned from the New Zealand experience. The following points can easily be applied to the current and new wave of health-care reforms across Canada.

- Recognize that sometimes hard decisions need to be made.
- Engage the public fully in the consultation process and be sincere.
- Appreciate that incremental change may not be sufficient.
- Never underestimate the role politics will play.
- Carefully determine the appropriate geographic scale in which new structures will be put in place.
- Ensure that everyone is "at the table" to design the new system.
- If integrated care is the primary goal, then design a structure that can facilitate this integration.
- It is essential to have political will and motivation.
- Acknowledge mistakes, learn from them and make appropriate changes.
- Ensure that evaluation is embedded in the process of health-care reform.

References

Health Policy. 1994. Vol. 29. Special Issue.

Lovelace, C. 1995. "A View from the Antipodes: NZ's Health Sector Reforms." Paper given at the 8th Annual CHEPA Conference, Toronto. May.

Salmond, G., M. Laugesen and K. Nelson. 1995. "Growing Pains or Enduring Tensions: Two Years into New Zealand Health Reforms." Wellington: Health Services Research Centre, Victoria University.

Southern Regional Health Authority, *Purchasing Directions, 1994/95 Summary.* 1994.

7

Lessons from Regionalization of Health Care in Canada

Saskatchewan

John Malcom

HEALTH REFORM

The Saskatoon District Health Board was formed in February 1992 as one of the first districts to be established in Saskatchewan. There are presently 30 districts in total with responsibility for acute, long-term care, home care, mental health, addiction, ambulance, and public health services. The Saskatoon District provides primary care to 225,000 people, regional care to the northern half of the province totalling half a million, and tertiary level services for the full population of 1,000,000. The district is the academic health centre for Saskatchewan with an affiliation with the University of Saskatchewan School of Medicine.

The budget for health services is $300 million with two-thirds being allocated to managed agencies and one-third directed towards affiliates in acute care and long-term care. The district has two rural hospitals that were converted to health centres, one in the late 1960s and the other in the fall of 1993.

WORKING TOGETHER

Health reform in Saskatchewan and in Alberta is based on virtually the same model. Interestingly, three of the four major urban districts, Saskatoon, Regina, and Calgary chose the same two words as the starting point in their motto. Saskatoon's motto is *"Working Together to Improve Health,"* and both Calgary and Regina have chosen *working together* as their first two words. In a recent article in the *New England Journal of Medicine*, John Iglehart, writing on the future of academic health centres, identified in the United States that "health care is transformed from a cottage industry to a more integrated business." Saskatchewan led the country in having cottage hospitals and the reform represents an integration of services in an effort to deliver the best possible services with reduced resources.

LESSONS

Accountability

The formation of districts has increased the accountability for health services. There are three specific areas where accountability is evident.

No excuses. Where in the past it was possible to "blame" another portion of the health system for inadequacy, districts are now responsible for the full range of services provided. For example, problems with long stays in hospitals awaiting placement in special care homes are traditionally blamed on the assessment function or inadequate resources in special care homes. In Saskatoon, this means that the district would be blaming itself since it has responsibility for both acute and long-term care. Over the past two years, we have been able to reduce the number of beds in our system being used by long stay patients from 50 to approximately ten, with our objective being zero when this represents an inappropriate placement for the individual.

Public interest. Over the past year, our district had 364 reports in the media. Not all were positive, not all were negative. The formation of the district has made it easier for the media to access a single location to obtain an immediate response on an issue. This is appropriate due to the rapid change being experienced in the delivery of services in our district and the interest the public has on its impact on services. This was one of the surprises that I discovered on accepting the job and I contacted a regional CEO in New Brunswick to see if they had also experienced a significant increase in media and public interest in what was happening, which was confirmed to be the case.

Evidence. As we have taken away the independence of organizations in order to promote the concept of an integrated system, it is important that we take the time to collect the information, evaluate the changes and demonstrate that these changes have, overall, been positive. It is not surprising that whenever you take something away from people, as is the case as we move to a systems approach away from an independent organizational cottage industry, that people will demand evidence as to its effectiveness. On the first week on the job, I was greeted with a letter in the paper claiming a significant increase in the number of administrative staff associated with the district.

The physician who wrote the letter had obtained a copy of the phone directory and added up the number of individuals involved, claiming that this was an addition to the administrative structure. The fact that a single directory had been produced highlighted the number of administrative people working in the district. Prior to formation of the district, these positions were hidden, in that not all hospitals, long-term care, public health and home care listed their administrative staff in a single location. Before the formation of the board, there were 24 senior staff in the organizations managed by the district, by the time reorganization had been completed in the fall of 1993, a total of 14 individuals filled the senior positions. The best example is our vice-president of finance, who was hired into health care by St. Paul's, accepted employment six months prior to the board's creation as the vice-president of finance for Royal University Hospital and presently has his office at Saskatoon City Hospital. When there were three independent hospitals, there were three V-Ps finance whereas now he performs that function on a systemwide basis.

Information

Nowhere was the cottage industry mentality more evident than in the collection and dissemination of information. In fact, I facetiously have said the only criteria on which information was collected prior to the formation of the board was that each site ensured that the information would be collected in a fashion that would not allow for comparison with peers in the community. The board started with virtually no integrated information systems and over the past three years has been faced with the development of both management and clinical information systems.

Imagine how successful credit cards would be if Visa said that you must have a different credit card for every site at which you purchase a product. Yet this is the experience we have with hospital registration cards. The one advantage of not having good integrated information systems was that it allowed the board to start afresh as it tried to identify what information is most appropriate. In collecting information,we have focused on three areas.

Population. Because we are a district with a variety of health-care services and priorities, the starting point in our data collection is with the total population we serve rather than on the basis of looking at it from a site-specific service perspective. Our district was also fortunate in that from day one, the responsibility for public health within the city of Saskatoon was included as part of the mandate. The public health/epidemiological approach to information has been a corner stone of our information systems with public health "acting as a conscience" for our health system.

Utilization. Our district has been able to undertake utilization audits that allow us to assess how we presently utilize our services. Audits have been completed systemwide on emergency services, critical care units and the operating suites. When faced with significant lay-offs of nurses last year, we took the opportunity to audit every Operating Room (OR) procedure being performed on all three sites in each theatre over a four-week period. This unique body of knowledge has allowed our OR committee to examine how best to utilize our OR services based on hard data, rather than relying upon the historical biases that may favour or detract from an individual site.

In addition, we have been fortunate that the Health Services Utilization and Research Commission has been active looking at how services are utilized on a provincial basis. The long-term care study, which was based on data made available through our Coordinated Assessment Unit, demonstrated that need for special care home placement ranked fourth in criteria determining the priority of admission to a special care home. After age, the most significant factor explaining admission was whether the individual was located in a residential apartment attached to a special care home. As a district, we are in a much better position to approach all of our affiliates, as well as our managed organizations, to say that we must change based on the evidence, rather than relying on historical preferences.

Efficiency. As a system we are also in a good position to examine the efficiency opportunities that exist from "best practices" that may be evident in each site. Why should we accept a higher unit cost on one site when the same service can be offered elsewhere at a lower cost?

Opportunity

Approaching issues from a systems point of view provides opportunities that may not be as easily achieved when examined on an individual site basis. For example, we have made progress in the following areas.

Quality. The creation of a districtwide medical staff with a large number of physicians practicing within most of the divisions has improved the quality of our peer review process. It also provides for the ability to learn of quality initiatives on one site and to transfer them relatively quickly to a second site.

Consumer centred. As we are a large organization, we are attentive to the fact that we not become more bureaucratic and have therefore tried to ensure that we simplify processes. We recognize that we have both internal and external consumers and that we need to improve processes for both.

Sustainability. The Canadian health-care system faces many challenges over the next few years. As a province, Saskatchewan has dealt with its

provincial deficit and now faces the impact of a second series of reductions associated with the Established Programs Funding reductions from
the federal government. While we do not look forward to this second round,
as a district we feel we are in a better position to deal with these reductions
in a fashion that will allow us to continue to deliver appropriate services.

New Brunswick

Russell King

INTRODUCTION

I am pleased to be able to share with you some of New Brunswick's experiences and lessons learned in dealing with a social imperative by now very familiar to most Canadians: health reform. It continues to pose ever greater challenges to those of us commited to ensuring our publicly-funded health system remains efficient, effective, and affordable.

One thing we knew from the outset: our efforts would come to nothing if we did not have a coordinated, comprehensive and integrated plan in place. And that plan could not work without system regionalization.

In detailing New Brunswick's unique approach to rationalizing, refocusing and restructuring its health and community service system, let me start by taking you back a little. In the spring of 1992, our government announced a major restructuring and rationalization of the province's hospital system.

This involved establishing regional hospital corporations to achieve multi-facility management throughout the entire province. It was part of the first stage of a two-stage, comprehensive reorientation of the entire health and community services system. Naturally, it became the focus of much attention from the Opposition parties, service providers, the media and the public.

The other main focal points of stage one included development and implementation of a physician resources plan, revisions to the provincial prescription drug program, increased funding for health promotion and disease prevention, expansion of ambulatory and in-home services, and improved ambulance services.

HISTORICAL CONTEXT FOR CHANGE

To give you some context for the health reform process in New Brunswick, it is important to know that in 1967 the government of New Brunswick fundamentally restructured itself. Known as Equal Opportunity, this initiative abolished county governments and centralized authority and responsibility for education, justice, welfare and housing, social services and health at the provincial level.

Since then, the government has played a key role in funding and service delivery, and has become the employer for public schools and hospital workers.

The minister of health was given broad regulatory powers, but individual hospital boards were retained and had considerable operational management authority.

In the late 1970s, the era of fiscal restraint began. The government slowly introduced measures to control costs, to more equitably distribute resources and services, and to improve operational effectiveness and efficiency. Hospitals also took measures to stretch their resources, including group purchasing of supplies.

A hospital system master plan defined the approved service base of each hospital. This was introduced to achieve a better planned and coordinated service network.

Progress was slow. Hospitals tended towards turf protection. Efforts to produce better regional and provincial planning were often viewed warily and sometimes openly opposed. Duplication of effort and overlap were common features of the system. As fiscal realities became more difficult, it became clearer that a fundamental restructuring of the entire system was necessary in order to improve efficiency and effectiveness, while maintaining a suitable level of patient-care services.

Studies as far back as 1969, and as recent as the McKelvey-Levesque Commission, created in the late 1980s by the current administration, recommended that government play a stronger leadership role in health-system design.

Following the presentation of the report by the McKelvey-Levesque Commission, our government began to reform the health-care system. It focused first on initiatives to improve the management of medicare, the

Prescription Drug Program, alternatives to institutional care, such as the Extra-Mural Hospital and improved out-patient space in conventional hospitals.

There was also an increased emphasis on health promotion and disease prevention.

THE PLAN

In late 1991, the Department of Health and Community Services was charged with the task of developing a comprehensive proposal for rationalizing and restructuring the system. In 1992, the government put in place a new governance and administrative structure for the province's hospital system.

On 25 March 1992, we announced the key elements of the plan. They included:

- the abolition of New Brunswick's individual hospital and health service centre facility boards;
- their replacement by eight regional hospital corporations (RHC) with the authority to operate all hospital and health service centre facilities in their region;
- administrative consolidation and establishment of regional medical staffs;
- revised roles for several of the 32 general hospitals, closure of nearly 300 beds, or 7 percent of the total, and conversion of four small hospitals to emergency/out-patient facilities (through these measures, the government's target ratio of five active treatment beds per 1,000 people was reached);
- expansion of the Extra-Mural Hospital to cover the remaining 20 percent of the province;
- expansion of the Single Entry Point (SEP) assessment and referral process for long-term care services;
- revision of the Hospital System Master Plan to more clearly define the service package for each hospital facility;

- introduction of the Physician Resource Plan, specifying supply and distribution targets for each region;
- consolidation of public sector funding for ambulance services, introduction of new vehicle, equipment and training standards, and the establishment of regional planning bodies; and
- the testing of a community health centre model in one community.

The new boards have 12 to 16 appointed, volunteer members, with the regional CEO and medical staff president as non-voting members. Representation on the board is based on the region's population distribution.

The minister makes four appointments, the board three, and the rest are generally appointed by groups of municipalities throughout the region. The boards select their own chairs and CEOs.

The board members, the chairs and the CEOs were all appointed by the minister for the first two years, since this was the transition period.

Responsibilities of regional hospital corporations include:

- internal organizational structure and operations;
- financial planning, budgeting and management;
- physician credentialling/granting of privileges;
- utilization management/quality assurance;
- maintaining established service quality and efficiency standards;
- internal bed and service distribution;
- human resource management;
- operational issues management;
- maintenance; and
- assuring effective working relationships with related organizations.

At the corporate management level, there is usually a staff complement of between seven and ten. This includes the region's CEO, senior managers covering key functions, and support staff.

At the facility level, there is usually a full-time, on-site administrator and managers. In some cases, it has proven effective for one person or a small team to administer more than one facility.

EFFECTS OF RESTRUCTURING

Initial reaction from small to medium sized hospital boards, local doctors, citizens' groups, the Catholic religious orders and the Opposition parties was often negative. Loss of jobs, civic pride and hospital beds being considered equivalent to "good care," were frequently cited as reasons to maintain the status quo.

The government presented its case in the Legislature, at "town hall" meetings, through media events, letters in the newspapers and speeches. Those who had basic disagreements, usually stakeholders, often remained sceptical. However, over time, the public has come to realize that predictions of lost services have simply not come true. But varying degrees of suspicion and resistance concerning government long-term plans still persist in some localities.

The positive results to date have been:

- a regional perspective on service rationalization and development planning has already been achieved;
- coordination and cooperation are now more evident and will continue to improve;
- functional and physical administrative consolidation have improved efficiency and reduced costs;
- greater emphasis on alternatives to in-patient care has been aided by bed closures, EMH expansion, SEP, enhanced Emergency and outpatient service capability, and better clinical utilization management;
- a provincial utilization management coordinating committee has been set up to provide a general framework, to monitor progress and address utilization issues on a systemwide basis;
- regional cancer committees have been established; and,
- regional computer compatibility has been achieved and an information bank is in place.

These and other benefits help to make better use of all available resources within the system, whether the public makes the connection or not.

I might note at this point that without regionalization, we would not have a physician resource plan. We have brought in further plans for nursing personnel and rehabilitation personnel. Regionalization facilitates management and target setting. It also helps take a coordinated approach to such things as trauma, treating the acutely ill, and ambulance services. We can establish common standards. Regionalization allows us to decentralize our efforts in a way that was impossible with competitive board structures at every hospital.

The untenable alternative to rationalization would have been to do nothing, let the inefficiencies continue and simply squeeze the system financially. That would have been irresponsible. Clearly, what was needed was a modernization of the system; one involving multi-facility governance with a consolidated administrative structure for each corporation that could improve overall efficiency and effectiveness without compromising service quality.

While we support regionalism, regionalism was not, and is not, our ultimate objective. We did not regionalize everything. We looked at what needed to be done, within the New Brunswick context, and proceeded to do it. Our hospital administration was regionalized. The Department of Health and Community Services was reorganized along the same geographic boundaries.

There is a debate as to whether it is an advantage to have all health and community services under one large board. Our regional hospital boards are focused on function, not advocacy.

Members are volunteers. The McKelvey-Levesque Report recommended that we establish regional health councils. However, we chose what I would call the "politically correct" approach: we simply said that hospitals cannot work in isolation. Now, as the regional corporations function as they were intended, and with departmental services delivered on a regional basis, we see all parts of the system working as a unit. We are establishing programs that cross divisional and departmental lines.

So, by functional design, we support regionalism as a logical way, in New Brunswick, to maintain a relevant, efficient, effective, accessible health system, without user fees.

IMPLEMENTATION

The implementation process for the new structure included:

- a new hospital act to replace the *Public Hospitals Act*;
- establishment of new RHCs;
- preparation for interim operational guidelines for RHCs;
- appointment of members and CEOs;
- preparation of model by-laws;
- discussions with RHCs regarding organization, funding, human resource and operational policy concerns;
- establishment of initial RHC organizational structure; and
- modification of the department's Hospital Services branch to relate more effectively with the new RHCs.

Implementation issues included:

- specific issues concerning the operation of Catholic hospitals;
- open or closed board meetings; and
- service rationalization between two hospitals in Saint John.

HEALTH REFORM: STAGE TWO

The second stage of health reform involved the introduction of a comprehensive long-term care strategy. The service network includes hospital extended care units, a portion of the EMH, nursing homes, special care homes, and community residences. It also includes reorganization of the family and community social services network, and a refocusing and restructuring of its programs and services.

A provincial physical rehabilitation services plan has been established to define the service roles of various agencies, and the operational links required to improve efficiency and effectiveness, as well as addressing human resource supply and distribution needs.

A nursing service resource and management plan has been set up that specifies supply and distribution requirements for nurses across the health-care system.

A new method of funding distribution for the hospital system has been devised, with hospital corporation input, and is being phased in to help improve equity and encourage sound clinical utilization management practices.

LESSONS LEARNED

One of the most important lessons we learned, and we learned it quickly during the reform process, was a political one. We attempted to depoliticize the system. This is much easier with an integrated plan such as the one driving health reform in New Brunswick. Having such a plan enables the government to deal more effectively with interest groups, associations, big and little "P" politics and placard wavers. They may not like the minister of the day, but the virtues of the plan are there — intact and visible. In streamlining New Brunswick's health and community services system, we found that, despite the temporary heat generated by some decisions, swift, decisive action is better than uncertainty and lack of direction.

This approach offers considerable opportunity to improve the use of existing resources and to increase productivity. This includes organization, management and the delivery of care. It allows for a greater percent of resources to go directly to patient care, while a lower percentage is expended on support services and administration.

With more comprehensive system planning, there is less risk of parochialism or "turf wars" because the regional hospital corporation concept provides a bigger picture regarding resource deployment.

A "bigger picture" approach makes it easier to deal with the issue of jobs within the system. It also provides better coordination of services and consequently improved organizational continuity. It means less time and effort need be spent on interorganizational debate and negotiation among single facility providers with competing agendas regarding local needs, demands, priorities and resource sharing — issues which may contradict the government's policy on the wise use of limited resources.

The RHC also allows for better clinical support from larger facilities for smaller ones. Health and medical professionals in smaller facilities are not as isolated because of improved access to services available at larger centres and being part of the region's clinical team.

As well, there is a greater potential for out-sourcing selected support services such as food, laundry, and housekeeping, due in part to economies of scale. It is also easier to realize the benefits of group purchasing both within and among regional corporations.

The regional corporation concept also helps improve the overall system management. It requires the government to be clear and consistent in its planning for system development and rationalization, to focus on a better measurement of expenditure outcomes, and to ensure the clear authority and accountability for the hospital corporations.

Without a regionalized approach to health reform, vital initiatives such as physician resource planning and the establishment of cancer committees would not be possible.

CONCLUSION

This is the context and a broad outline of the health-reform process we have developed, and continue to implement, in New Brunswick. We believe it is an evolutionary, progressive attempt to modernize our system of health and community social services. We also believe it must be done regardless of the present need for restraint.

The ultimate good of health reform, for any jurisdiction, is to ensure that services and programs remain relevant and responsive to public need, and that they continue to be delivered efficiently, effectively and affordably.

Quebec

Paul A. LaMarche

INTRODUCTION

I would like to stress the following four points in this paper: (i) the reasons for pursuing decentralization in the management of health care in Quebec; (ii) the form of decentralization adopted; (iii) the point Quebec has now reached and the results obtained so far; and (iv) the lessons learned.

REASONS FOR FURTHER DECENTRALIZATION OF MANAGEMENT OF THE QUEBEC HEALTH-CARE SYSTEM

There were four reasons why Quebec had decided to pursue the decentralization of its health-care system. The first was the conviction that the problems facing the Quebec health-care system, particularly the lack of adaptability of the services to the needs and characteristics of the population and the relative effectiveness with which resources were used, was due in part to the overcentralization of decisionmaking: the Ministry of Health and Social Services.

The ministry had to decide on each request sent in by over 900 health and social services institutions, over 1,500 community organizations, and a large number of professional groups. For example, the ministry had to decide which of two competing hospitals should acquire axial tomography capability in a remote region where half would have been sufficient to meet the demands of the population; which of three competing hospitals should obtain a pediactric centre in a region where the birth rate has dropped drastically over the last decade; whether nursing homes or home care should be given the money for providing care to the same elderly persons in the same small community.

It became obvious that the ministry could not know the needs and the preferences of the people better than the people themselves. It was much less well-acquainted with the performance of health resources than the people affected by them and those closest to the real action.

The second reason was that there was no democratic forum for debating and choosing from the numerous requests coming from a multitude of interest groups acting in health care: a forum that the population could identify with; a forum that the population could have the sense of being able to influence; a forum that the population could believe in.

The third reason was the perception by several regions that the central authority had the tendency to decide mainly in favour of large urban centres, like Montreal and Quebec, and not to take sufficiently into account the specific characteristics of other regions.

The fourth reason was a growing political identification with one's own region and the growing feeling that the region would be better served if the people had the opportunity to decide for themselves.

THE FORM OF DECENTRALIZATION

In Quebec, decentralization has aimed to bring decisionmaking closer to the action. In doing so, it has put the decisionmaking and accountability in the hands of those to whom care is provided and who would pay the cost no matter the form — that is, the people. In Quebec, decentralization, democratization, and accountability of decisionmaking go hand in hand.

To decentralize decisionmaking, Quebec decided to transform its previous Health and Social Services Regional Councils into regional boards. While regional councils were essentially advisory in nature, regional boards are executive and decisionmaking bodies.

Quebec divided its territory into 18 regions, each headed by a regional board. Regional boards fulfil five main functions. The first one is to identify the health and well-being priorities of their region. These priorities should not be defined in terms of services to be provided or resources to be obtained, but rather in terms of health and social problems facing their population that should be tackled in order of priority. The second is the elaboration of regional service plans to address these health and social priorities. These plans should not be limited to the contribution of health care and social services but should also include the contribution of other sectors in addressing these problems. The third is the allocation of financial resources to health and social service institutions as well as to volunteer and non-governmental organizations involved in health and social services. To this end regional boards are to receive a global financial envelope based on the population to be served and on its characteristics rather than on the number of producers in the region and the cost of the services produced. This financial envelope does not include, however, physicians' fees.

The last two functions are to undertake public health measures, to ensure the efficient use of resources, and to evaluate the effectiveness of the services provided.

To democratize the decisionmaking process, several measures have been taken: giving lay people the majority of seats on the boards of directors of each health and social service institution and regional board; selecting the people sitting on boards from those residing in the region; having the people sitting on boards elected either by electoral colleges or directly by the people themselves during annual assemblies; making boards of directors' meetings open to the public; and reserving a question period for the public at all boards of directors meetings.

Mechanisms have been designed to ensure dual accountability: first to those being served and second to those paying. All institutions must have an annual public meeting during which they must provide information about the previous year's decisions and must respond to questions from the floor, including from the media. All institutions are reviewed by regional boards during public audiences regarding both the services provided and the use of resources. All boards of governors of regional boards must have their annual report endorsed by their regional assembly. Regional assemblies are microcosms of repesentatives of regional groups with a strong interest in health and social services. It is these regional assemblies that elect the boards of directors of regional boards.

Finally, at least every three years, each regional board must appear before the Parliamentary Commission on Social Affairs concerning both the services to the population and the use of resources. Hearings at local and regional levels must occur before hearings at the provincial level. The expectation was that everything which had been raised at local and regional levels and had not been resolved, would come up at the provincial level to be discussed, debated, and hopefully resolved.

Thus, in Quebec, decentralization and democratization of both decisionmaking and accountability go hand in hand.

THE EXTENT OF IMPLEMENTATION OF DECENTRALIZATION AND THE RESULTS OBTAINED SO FAR

The health-care reform, launched in 1991, was intended to change only three aspects of the Quebec health-care system: the objectives; the decisionmaking; and a few rules of the game.

So far, we have succeeded in shifting the objectives of our health-care system from increasing accessibility to quality care to outcome-oriented objectives; that is, specific health and social problems to be solved. We have succeeded in shifting accessibility to quality care from an objective to a means. A Health and Well-being Policy was adopted by the Government of Quebec. This policy identified 19 specific health and social problems to be tackled in order of priority by our health and social services system.

After the adoption and publication of this policy, each region was requested to identify its own health and well-being priority problems. There have been three quite interesting results of the regional priority process: all the regions focused on the same six problems; those six problems were related more to the quality of life than to the causes of death. They concern negligence, abuse, and violence towards the young, the elderly, and women; behavioural problems among youth; substance abuse; mental health problems, including suicide; social integration of the elderly; and cancer and cardiovascular diseases. The third result was the obvious and considerable gap between the priority problems and the actual allocation of resources.

If there is one major positive result of the Quebec reform, so far, it is that finally the system is focusing on people's health and social problems rather than on services to be developed or the resources to be obtained. The main challenge now is how to link resource allocation with the main health and well-being service problems. Priorities seem to be more useful, at present, for writing speeches than for allocating resources.

We have also succeeded in changing the decisionmakers. All boards of directors were modified to allow more room for lay people. We consider the election process of boards of directors a great success. More than 7,000 people came forward for the election to the 1,200 available seats. More than 170,000 people participated in these elections.

There has been some success — albeit to a limited extent — in democratizing the decisionmaking process. On the positive side, meetings of regional boards of directors attract, on average, between 100 and 200 people in each region. I have seen meetings of 500 people in the audience. The more problems there are in a region, the more people are attending the meetings of boards of directors. Time has been allowed for public questions. Meetings of boards of directors are now covered by the media so that the debates that are going on in health and health care, and the decisions that have to be made, are more and more open to the public.

On the negative side, however, some boards of governors have not been composed of lay people to the extent envisaged. Health professionals and representatives of health institutions succeeded in being elected through different electoral colleges with the result that certain regional boards are composed of almost 50 percent health professionals. Some boards of directors hold two meetings: the real one, behind closed doors, and the one for the public. The bureaucracy of some regional boards acts as if lay people on boards of governors are a nuisance rather than representatives of the people they are there to serve. But overall, it is agreed in Quebec that the decisionmaking process has been more democratic since the reform than it was before, although some improvements are still needed.

One main problem resides in changing the rules of the game — mainly the allocation of resources. In the beginning, regional financial envelopes were to be transferred to regional boards a maximum of 18 months after their creation. It was later decided that the transfer of the allocation of resources would occur only in 1998. The point in time at which resource allocation would be transferred from the ministry to the regions seems to be postponed by one year every year.

What we are now realizing, although we suspected it all along, is that changing the health-care system objectives and the decisionmaking process was not challenging the role of the Ministry of Health and Social Services. Changing the rules of the game, particularly concerning the allocation of resources, does. This is where the most resistance is felt.

LESSONS TO BE LEARNED FROM THE QUEBEC DECENTRALIZATION PROCESS

Five lessons could be learned from the Quebec experience. The first one is that decentralization is good and is needed, but for someone else, not for oneself. Every health and social service organization advocated decentralization as a means to solving the problems that face our system while simultaneously advocating that they should continue to be answerable to a central authority because of their own distinct characteristics. Teaching hospitals, private institutions, and community organizations all stressed the need for decentralization in general. But each also pointed out their own particularities to maintain direct links with the ministry.

The second is that regional boards could in fact constitute democratic fora for decisionmaking. But they could also disguise themselves as ministries of health centralizing the decisionmaking at the regional level and bureaucratizing the decisionmaking process. The last thing that Quebec needs at present is 18 ministries of health and social services.

The third lesson is that putting the structure into place is one thing, but having all the relevant actors play according to the new rules is another. More time is needed to assess the extent to which these new rules will be implemented to produce the expected results.

Lesson number four is that the process of decentralization could be caught in a "catch-22" situation. In our system, decentralization requires the co-operation of a central authority. But, the main resistance to decentralization comes from the central authority who is likely to lose power and influence through decentralization.

Three types of resistance are manifested by the Ministry of Health. The first one is the postponing of transfers of important functions to the regional boards. The allocation of resources is a good example. The second, and a more subtle one, is that mechanisms that were designed to ease decentralization are becoming instruments of detailed control on the part of the ministry. Approval of regional service plans by the ministry is a good example. The third method of resistance is not making a transfer of staff to correspond to the transfer of new functions to the regions.

The fifth and final lesson is that no matter what the form or process of decentralization, final public accountability remains in the hands of the minister of health and social services. Until decentralization has been coupled with a universal ballot and taxation, central accountability provides the necessary and sufficient excuse for interfering with the decisionmaking process at the regional level.

Ontario

Alan Warren

It is inevitable that after nearly 20 years service with the District Health Council in Ottawa-Carleton, I approach the topic of regionalization and decentralization with the Ontario DHC experience in mind. I shall, in the course of this paper, share my thoughts on the good and bad features of the DHC concept, and touch on prospects for regionalization in the future in Ontario. I do not intend to discuss projects which are sometimes described as forms of regionalization but which are really hospital merger or rationalization exercises. The much publicized Windsor Project is an example. This is not a regionalization initiative.

The topic is of interest nationally because of the variety of approaches adopted across Canada and internationally because of the structural variations to be found in the health-care systems of other jurisdictions. Comparisons are inescapable. I would emphasize and re-emphasize that the evaluation of experience elsewhere is critical to the next steps we take in Ontario.

As many others have noted, there is confusion not only about regionalization as a concept but in the terms used. Such words as devolution, decentralization, deconcentration, and delegation are used interchangeably with the term regionalization. This, in some ways, is reflected in the regionalization (or "districtization") which has been introduced across the country. The degree to which authority or responsibility has been allocated varies considerably, although the intent seemed at one time to be devolution with broad powers, but this is now being questioned. At the root of the issue, however, as it will apply to Ontario, is the basic question: What should constitute a region in population and/or geographic terms?

In Ontario — apart from a brief flirtation in 1969 by the then Ontario Council of Health — regionalization of the health-care system has not been explored with any conviction or consistency. Although we have had, for many years, six recognized planning regions based on early referral patterns related to health-science centres, the most significant initiative was the development of our District Health Councils. The concept was devised by the Ontario Council of Health in 1973 via the Mustard Report. To this extent Ontario was in the forefront of decentralization or delegation of responsibilities. But the responsibilities delegated were limited and the new DHCs were defined as "advisory." Setting aside reservations about the size of the districts and therefore boundaries (which have never been seriously questioned since the introduction of the DHCs) the concept was good, even bold for the times. The objective was to conduct planning and priority-setting at a local level where community needs and values could best be taken into account. The councils were also to plan comprehensively, a challenge none could fully meet, given the scale of the system, the freedoms exercised within it, and the blurring of the health-care sector into others sectors such as social services.

The composition of the councils was important — a mix of consumers, providers, and local (elected) municipal representatives in a 40-40-20 percent split. This has stood the test of time. The councils were expected to provide advice to the minister (and to his/her officials), but the more enlightened communities quickly saw that a DHC should also give advice to the community it served, including its provider agencies and the municipality. The associated roles of interpreter (of policies as well as needs) and broker-arbitrator then became evident. These both are good and important features which are even today not always appreciated.

The worst feature of this new concept, in my view, was that its introduction was voluntary and protracted, a reflection perhaps of Ontario's well-known caution and incrementalism. Although ministry staff allocated to the task worked diligently to promote the DHC concept, lead citizens in the various districts had to take the initiative, to convince local politicians, citizens, and providers of the potential value of a DHC. They had to propose the formation of a DHC to the minister, who then approved its establishment and named its members.

In the mid-1970s, when the views of providers prevailed, this was thought to be the appropriate way to introduce change. The result was that it has taken over 20 years to develop the full network of DHCs across the province.

The consequent variance in experience and achievement has made it extremely difficult to establish the DHC "movement" with the overall credibility it needs, and has weakened its potential for evolution. This lack of development or evolution is one of the negative features of the DHC experience. Now, while the health-care system is subject to scrutiny and restructuring, DHCs are apparently expected to go serenely on, basically unchanged in role and structure since their introduction in 1973.

On the other hand, the freedom of initiative and flexibility which was allowed to DHCs in the early years, features that made them attractive, has given way to increasing control and direction from the Ministry of Health, to the point where some observers have expressed the view that DHCs are now little more than branch offices of the ministry, a trend that runs counter to other experiences across the country. While standards must be set by the ministry and DHC performances evaluated, the increasing detail of directives (e.g., the precise definition of a DHC committee structure and composition) must be listed as one of the less acceptable aspects of present day DHCs.

As more DHCs were formed the ministry's internal structure had to adjust to accommodate the DHCs' activities and information needs. The ministry, however, has not been uniform in its attitude to the DHCs, with some branches and divisions being more inclined to collaborate than others. The ambivalence suggests a resistance, conscious or otherwise, to the transfer of any degree of power from an established bureaucracy.

In 1989 an attempt was made by Deputy Minister Martin Barkin to broaden the activities of the DHCs, perhaps to reinvigorate them and make them more supportive of the ministry as it faced the necessity of change to the system. A so-called "expanded role" was announced, building on the original, very broad, terms of reference but still leaving the DHCs in a purely advisory role. For the record, the four areas of enhancement were (i) allocation of funds; (ii) district human resource planning; (iii) strengthening area-wide planning; (iv) and integration of health and social service planning.

The limited additional staff resources that were made available, coupled with continued, studied avoidance of the question of the transfer of any degree of real authority, has meant that the expanded role has not been developed properly in any of the four areas. However, councils generally have made progress in area-wide (regional) consultative planning; in fact, their regional orientation and cooperation was evident long before the official enhancement statement. The regional planning occurs through regular and task-oriented interdistrict meetings within the six recognized regions. But I stress that this is interdistrict, cooperative planning and like every other aspect of the work of DHCs, is advisory.

One region, however, the southwest, after an abortive attempt to establish a fully devolved system in 1991 (the Orser Report) embarked on another attempt to put some teeth into regional planning in 1993 with the intent of devising a model or mechanism to achieve that aim. A report and recommendation was issued in mid-1994 and the model, which envisages a Regional Health Council funded and staffed as a distinct entity, received the support of the minister of health, and I understand is poised to begin its operations. The Regional Council is to draw its membership from each of the DHCs in the region, together with representatives of the Academic Health Sciences in that region.

Critics see this model as another layer in a planning system that needs overhaul, a model that does little to resolve the issues of authority and accountability. It is a mechanism seemingly not favoured in the other regions in the province and thus must be seen as a "pilot" or an exploratory test of DHC evolution. The question of the authority of the Regional Council is unavoidable. If its conclusions have to be endorsed individually by all DHCs in the region, the scene is set for delay, frustration, and compromise. In the final analysis, nothing is gained in comparison with the more informal inter-DHC regional planning. If the Regional Council is to be given planning authority over the DHCs why stop there, if this to be a demonstration or pilot?

The time has surely come for the Ontario government to recognize that its Ministry of Health cannot manage, effectively, a highly complex health-care system serving over 11 million people. The province needs to be divided into more manageable parcels, with the appropriate degree of authority and funding control transferred to authorities serving those parcels. Once the decision to decentralize or devolve is made, two questions will present themselves. One, are these parcels to be described as regions as we seem to understand the term, (a population and/or geographic definition), or are they to be defined as managed care units? Two, in either case, what should be the size of the region or managed care unit, in population terms?

Popular theory, until recently, has suggested that a region in health-care terms needs to be 90 to 95 percent self-sufficient in services and resources. According to which authority you refer to, this can equate with a population figure ranging from 0.5 to 1.5 million people. In practice, internationally, you will find considerable variance and if you consider some American managed care organizations, you can find enrolled population groups (surrogate regions) much larger. Regions and managed care units can also be readily identified which are much smaller in service population (in Saskatchewan, for example), but such organizations need to pool resources or to engage in service purchasing from others, an administrative complication and possibly an additional inconvenience for patients.

I have introduced the topic of managed care deliberately as we have some limited experience with it in Ontario, under the title Comprehensive Health Organizations (CHOs). They are a form of devolution if not actual regionalization. A very large proportion of the American population is now enrolled with managed care organizations with, reportedly, significant success at cost containment and reduction of unnecessary service provision. In the United Kingdom the health-care system is moving quite rapidly in the same direction, at the expense of the established regional structures.

It is argued that there is no straightforward prescription for the regionalization of health care in Ontario because of its diversity, its uneven population distribution and its geography and that therefore a single model is going to be difficult to devise and apply. However, we have the recognized health planning regions to which I have referred and we already have regions and areas for the administration of social services. There are lessons to be learned from this experience, but Ontario also needs to learn from the successes and mistakes of other jurisdictions — nationally and internationally.

What is apparent is that if and when devolution or decentralization occurs, the structure will need to be newly devised, certainly incorporating the planning and negotiating skills and accumulated experience of DHCs, but I do not see them evolving into new regional authorities even if groups of DHCs were willing to merge. If the system evolves more into one based on managed care units, DHCs would be even less able to adapt. They have not been organized and "resourced" to manage even part of the system, and a change in role and orientation to management would be so massive as to equate to a new structure.

As I have noted, the single greatest weakness of the DHC concept was that the councils were created haphazardly over an extraordinary period of time and the real lesson for the next stage of development for Ontario's health-care system is that any regionalization should be done decisively and comprehensively, notwithstanding the issue of diversity. If the province could get it more or less right the first time, that would be a bonus and an example to the world.

On the other hand, noting the long experience and current trends in the United Kingdom system, it could be that by the time Ontario acts on regionalization, the pendulum will have swung again and the concept fallen out of favour.

8

The Human Realities of Regionalization

Roundtable Discussion

This roundtable, moderated by Dr. Jonathan Lomas, had spokespersons representing various interests:

Payer Representatives

Hon. Russell King (Provincial)
Terry Sullivan (Third-Party Payer)

Provider Representatives

Geoffrey Higgins M.D. (Physicians)
Carol Clemenhagen (Hospitals)

Consumer Representatives

Fiona Chin-Yee (Nova Scotia Health Action Coalition)
Stephen Learey (Canadian Health Coalition)

Each set of representatives offered a short presentation. These were followed by discussion and questions from the audience.

PAYER PERSPECTIVE

Russell King, in his opening remarks, observed that in representing the "payers," they were also providing input from the overall design aspect of the health system — two elements that were closely related. It had to be recognized that regionalization is essentially a tool used to maintain the health-care system and to avoid the duplication of resources, so that the system would work better, with a commonality of purpose.

Dr. King's Remarks

Commitment to Change. I believe that the status quo is not good enough, and I have a strong belief that change is necessary and will be of benefit in the long run. The McKelvey-Levesque Commission on Selected Health Care Programs clearly reinforced this view and added that we needed to be more forward in our thinking; that the status quo was not good enough for the people of New Brunswick. Change had to happen. Escalating costs were, of course, a factor. But like any organization (or individual), as a responsible consumer, you ask: What am I getting for the price I am paying? We need to examine our system critically.

System Approach. A whole vocabulary has been invented to describe what many organizations are trying to do — terms like re-engineering, restructuring, right-sizing. These words suggest that we are reviewing and reworking how systems have been organized. In New Brunswick, we have taken a "systems" approach to health and community services. The questions that have been asked by, for example, the McKelvey-Levesque Commission are: What is the existing system? What are the components of the system? What works and what does not seem to be working? How much does it cost? And most importantly, who should the system serve?

Health and community services are intended to meet human needs in many areas. They are humanitarian services. What price can you put on access and distribution of services? In theory, we can all say "whatever it costs, it's worth it," but in our world, there are limitations.

The health and community services system is too important to New Brunswickers. The challenge to develop and manage the system is real.

Changes to the system will have an impact on the lives of individuals and communities. Committed and caring service providers are concerned that these impacts are not all negative. We have to change our thinking and recognize that there are real limits to what the sytem can pay for. And we have to communicate that message.

We also — and perhaps this is most important — we have to start asking what are we achieving; what results do we want?

Determinants of Health. We have to take a broad look at what are the determinants of health. We have been listening to many views expressed in a variety of forums. For example, the Federal/Provincial and Territorial Advisory Committee on Population Health prepared a report for ministers entitled *Strategies for Population Health: Investing in the Health of Canadians* (September 1994). The overall role of the advisory committee is to advise the Conference of Deputy Ministers on National and International Strategies what should be pursued to improve the health status of the Canadian population and to provide a more integrated approach to health.

A population health approach differs from traditional medical and health-care thinking in two major ways. First, population health strategies address the entire range of factors that determine health; second, traditional health care focuses on risks and clinical factors related to particular diseases.

Population health strategies are designed to affect the entire population. Health care deals with individuals one at a time, usually individuals who already have a health problem or are at significant risk of developing one. In looking at the health-care system and the need for change, we had to consider which services have a positive impact on the well-being of New Brunswickers. We were very aware that changes to the health-care system would affect individuals and service provider groups.

Health is More than the Health-Care System. This has been a constant theme throughout the change process. We are concerned about the determinants of health — recognizing that health services are an important element to promote, maintain and restore health. But there are other factors that influence the health status of people.

I want to mention a couple of initiatives that affect people and illustrate our thinking. The Single Entry Point Program is now a provincewide program. It began as a pilot project in April 1989, and was developed after consultation with key stakeholders. The goal of the pilot project was to reduce the premature institutionalization of seniors who, with additional help and services, could continue to live at home. The Single Entry Point Model is based on the existence or establishment of a continuum of services capable of meeting different kinds of needs. The model focuses on solving the problem presented by the person requiring assistance, and involves the use of a multidisciplinary team who then assesses the individual.

Another major initiative is the Early Childhood Initiative (August 1993) which is intended to improve the life chances of children in New Brunswick by providing services to preschool children who are identified as at-risk because of physical, intellectual, and emotional disabilities or delays and because of family environments with a number of risk factors. As with the Single Entry Point Program, the service delivery model uses multidisciplinary teams with a range of services that focuses on the child. These services involve enhanced prenatal screening and intervention, including a nutrition intervention and supplement program; enhanced postnatal screening and intervention, including a nutrition supplement program; retargeted preschool health clinics (children three and a-half years of age); home-based intervention services; integrated daycare services; and social work prevention services.

There is increasing evidence that intervening at critical stages in the development of children and youth has the greatest potential for positively influencing their later health and well-being.

Our focus is on the client and the needs of the client, in order for him or her to function to their full potential. It is forward thinking — intended to provide an appropriate service at an appropriate time.

Management of Change Process. Once it was clearly understood that change was needed and that the signals had gone out that we were looking at health from a broad perspective, we also had to demonstrate that we had the fortitude to withstand criticism. We recognized that working with key stakeholders would be necessary in order to develop a system that would be both efficient and effective in the long term. We recognized the importance of clear, concise communication of our goals. There was and will continue to be a certain amount of resistance.

Management of Health Human Resources. The management of human resources is a fundamental aspect of health-care services. Human resources need to be relevant to the health needs of the population. Recognizing the critical role played by the physician in the health-care system, one of our first challenges was to look at physician resources. The Physicians Resources Advisory Committee developed a management plan which will enable New Brunswick to have, over the long term, a supply of physicians with training and specializations to deliver services to citizens. It is a plan that involves targets and recruitment incentives.

Nursing services are also a critical aspect of health care. Significant decisions on the part of the Nurses Association of New Brunswick led to the requirement of a Bachelor of Nursing as the entry level for practicing nurses. This decision has implications for the health-care system as well as nursing services. The concept of nursing services includes more than just nurses. Registered nursing assistants play an important role in the provision of nursing services. A Nursing Services Plan has been developed by an advisory committee which includes representatives of the Nursing Association, the Nurses' Union and the Association of New Brunswick Registered Nursing Assistants.

As with the physicians, it has not been easy to bring about agreement. There are implications for the membership of the various associations. There is anxiety and concern about job opportunities and job loss, about education and training opportunities, about scope of practice, and about the long-term impact of change on the professions and the population.

The Rehabilitation Services Plan (April 1994) is in the early stages of implementation. The primary goal of the plan is systematically to guide the development of a coordinated regionalized system of institutional and community-based rehabilitation services to meet the changing needs of New Brunswickers. While the primary providers of rehabilitation services are audiologists, occupational therapists, physiotherapists, and speech language pathologists, important roles are played by other formal and informal caregivers.

We identified the need for trained rehabilitation support personnel working under the direction of a rehabilitation professional. We have been working with the community college system and the rehabilitation professional associations to determine the functions of rehabilitation support persons and the type of training required to be able to do those functions. Again, this has not been an easy exercise.

Conclusion. The restructuring of the health-care system involves rethinking how and what we do and considering alternatives to the traditional patterns of service delivery and professional training. Change is not easy. It is stressful. We are moving into uncharted waters. We have tried to work with those groups and organizations that are likely to be most significantly affected by change. We also need to be steadfast in our purpose and not easily dissuaded. Unpopular decisions have had to be made. We know that we cannot please everyone — but we are committed to having a health-care system that serves the best interests of New Brunswickers. To do this, we have to develop and manage a cost-effective system of services.

When we step back and look at our restructuring efforts, we have achieved a lot in a short time. We recognize that change is an evolutionary process. The need to continue to review and revamp and reconsider what and how we do things as part of our environmental thinking. Communicating our intentions, clearly articulating what it is we feel we must do, meeting with stakeholders and individuals on an ongoing basis is critical to the process of change.

There are many "human realities" to the health-care system. Individuals, families, formal and informal caregivers, all play a significant role in the health and well-being of people.

Terrence Sullivan noted that the regional approaches developing in the provinces appeared to be concentrating on the coordination and rationalization of hospital services. Thus, particular attention was being paid to only one of the three key "cost drivers," that is, hospital beds, physician services, and technology. He proposed, therefore, to deal with the other two areas — physician services (human resources) and the assessment of technology and utilization management approaches.

Terrence Sullivan's Remarks

The first issue turns on how one can reasonably plan and budget for local health services regionally if all of primary care is coordinated from a centrally bargained, centrally administered provincial fee pool. Much of the specialty care dollars will be centrally administered as well, but the judicious use of admission privileges and hospital management techniques may play a useful role in the equitable development and dispersion of specialty care. In other words, if the majority of funds for physician services are centrally administered, it is challenging to see from a second- or third-party payer perspective how a regional structure can effectively influence the delivery of primary care. I seem to recall that Quebec at one time had an incentive/disincentive plan for underserviced/overserviced areas of primary care. With that exception, unless I am missing developments in other provinces, primary care remains a largely untouched issue in regionalization. Major labour force adjustments are going on in local health labour markets involving nurses, technical, and maintenance personnel, among others. In the dramatic labour force adjustments occurring in the health sector, only physicians maintain employment security. All the while the *supply and compensation of primary care physician services remain centrally managed.*

From the perspective of the "human face" of regionalization, there is little by way of coordinated linking of the labour market adjustment issues faced by "downsizing" and the role of regional labour market instruments in responding to these plans. For anyone who pretends to be interested in the social and economic determinants of health, employment and labour market adjustments are employment-planning considerations. In Ontario, the Ontario Training and Adjustment Board is not sufficiently well linked to the restructuring which is going on at the local or regional level in the health field. *A stronger link between regional health planning and management and labour market training and adjustment needs to be built.* There is and will continue to be major labour adjustment problems in this labour-intensive industry. Currently, there is no way of ensuring that hospital workers laid off in the restructuring are retrained for a revitalized community care sector, for example.

The final issue is whether we opt for a central versus regional approach to *technology*, in the larger sense of technology (i.e., effective investigation and treatment methods). Will regional structures provide different incentives to advance effective treatments and discourage ineffective treatments, or will they rely on provincial level utilization review mechanisms such as HSURC in Saskatchewan and the Guidelines Commission in British Columbia? We are facing this issue currently with respect to the management of back problems where there is no effective regional lever to discourage the unnecessary and costly x-rays of the low lumbar region apart from the long and labour-intensive journey of "physician education." From a third-party payer perspective, there is a temptation to recommend provincewide non-insurance for certain procedures or add authorization hurdles for such procedures. However, there may be some benefit for *competitive and innovative approaches to utilization management at the regional levels*.

PROVIDER PERSPECTIVE

It was asserted, at the outset, that there was a need to have effective provider input into regionalization, since this would have far reaching consequences for the health-care system, that is, beyond institutions to the family practitioner's office. *Dr. G. Higgins* proposed to deal with the need for effective input by providers.

Geoffrey Higgins' Remarks

One of the key stated objectives of regionalization has been to increase the role of what has been termed the citizen or consumer in health-care decisionmaking, both by directly increasing the representation of lay community members on regional boards and by moving the decisionmaking process closer to the community through the introduction of the regional boards themselves.

As regionalized structures have been introduced, however, there have been explicit attempts, in some jurisdictions, to exclude or minimize the participation and input of health-care providers, particularly at the board level but also among the many committees and working groups that advise the boards. This is done, in part, to avoid a direct conflict of interest situation, but also because of the perception that providers will promote their own self-interests and oppose any fundamental change in the organization of health care that might impinge upon those interests. Concern has been expressed that health-care providers cannot see the "big picture."

While encouraging broader representation from the community on regional boards is a laudable objective, I believe that it is important to have provider input for at least two reasons. First, health-care providers have always had a role to play in advocating for the provision of quality care by virtue of their specialized knowledge and by their direct contact with patients. This is a role that medical advisory committees and professional advisory committees have played very effectively over the years. This is a view that is shared by the public. In a survey of Canadian adults conducted by the Environics Research Group in the Spring of 1994, when asked who should be primarily responsible for making decisions such as buying "high-tech" equipment for a hospital or expanding public health programs, 61 percent said health professionals/administrators, while 19 percent said people in the local communities and 5 percent said elected politicians.

Second, we must remember that health human resources are the largest single component of the health service industry. It seems only reasonable that health-care workers should have the opportunity to provide input to the decisionmaking processes that directly affect their professional activities and working conditions.

I would like to briefly address the above two concerns. First, there is the question of whose interests are represented on the boards. Who is a typical representative of the community? There is always going to be an element of self-selection by interested parties, however boards are to be constituted. For example, the results of some "deliberative" polling conducted by the Centre for Health Economics and Policy Analysis (CHEPA) at McMaster University show widely varying levels of personal willingness with regard to specific decisionmaking activities such as planning and priority-setting, revenue raising, and distributing funds.

The preliminary results of further survey work by CHEPA demonstrate clearly that the composition of devolved authorities, to date, tends to be drawn much more heavily from the most highly educated and upper income brackets in the community as well as from among those with previous community board experience.

To me, this underscores the importance of assuring that recruitment to regional boards must be done through a clearly specified appointment or electoral process, one that includes explicit terms of reference for the participation of board members. Health-care providers should not be excluded from serving on regional boards, especially if there is an open electoral process. It is essential that they be represented on board committees and working groups.

When seeing the "big picture," I believe it is incumbent on us as health providers to equip ourselves with the necessary skills to participate effectively in regionalization, including issues of governance, needs assessment, health economics, evidence-based decisionmaking, and concepts of population health. There are a range of opportunities to do so, including undergraduate and graduate programs in health administration and business administration offered at several universities across Canada, the Health Services Management Program offered by the Canadian Hospital Association and the Physician Manager Institute of the Canadian Medical Association.

I would hope that as regionalization continues that issues of board composition and participation would be addressed in any evaluation framework that is applied.

Carol Clemenhagen's Remarks

I have been asked to make some remarks about the human realities of health-care providers in implementing regionalized models of health-service delivery.

Herman Crewson, a long-time participant in the Canadian health-care system, most recently retired as Head of the British Columbia Health Association, remarked when speaking about the health reform initiatives of this decade: "both taxpayers and consumers of health services will be beneficiaries of reform. It is the providers and funders that will have to adjust to the new realities — some with great difficulty."

Reform has provided growth opportunities for providers and has also created scenarios of personal loss as the health-care workplace is rationalized, re-directed, and reduced.

I would like to comment briefly on the type of health provider who will flourish in this high-impact environment and then go into a few of the human resource issues that have accompanied the move to regionalization.

What is needed in persons assuming front-line roles in reform? What is the survival kit of the nineties? The modern day management survival kit might well be innovativeness, the ability to sustain relationships, communication skills, and great flexibility. There is no neat recipe card for innovation — ignoring conventional boundaries and figuring out how to apply new ideas in the real world. The capacity to innovate may well be the single most important and elusive factor in health-care leadership.

Today's health-system providers must also be good negotiators and consensus builders, able to create a sustainable and sustaining network of colleagues, with a management team that includes medical staff leaders across regional settings. George Annas from Boston University has used an ecological metaphor to describe the new health-care leadership in contrast to the more militaristic themes that we may traditionally use to describe leaders. He speaks of a health system that is renewable and balanced, a system with limited resources that requires conservation and community support.

I hardly need to mention the importance of communicate! communicate! communicate! In all likelihood, 98 percent of all information can be shared. Certainly, by providing information on downsizing and lay-offs as soon as possible, the terrible anxiety of uncertainty is minimized. One of the sources of frustration for CEOs at the start of a regionalization process is that often they do not know any more than their employees about what is going to happen and they have a real sense of letting their people down by not being able to share any useful information that could ease tension levels.

The Ability to Adapt, or Flexibility Rounds out the Survival Kit. Flexibility is the ability to take on new roles and new responsibilities in areas outside earlier training and past experience. The interest and willingness to self-examine and redesign care practices in clinical situations is an example of the new leadership skill mix.

The management literature is full of overwrought and overworked analogies such as "surfing on the edge" — constantly adjusting, never falling, standing on the edge of a cliff and enjoying the view. I think we all have a bit of vertigo these days, precipitated by the realization that health care is expected to do its share and more in the deficit reduction fiscal agenda that all governments are now following.

The realities of the workplace today are that the workforce is downsized and less new workers enter, while it is aging. This may mean some loss of vibrancy, optimism, and new ideas that new people bring to any workforce. The opportunities for new graduates are clearly very limited.

Regionalism Has Meant not just Fewer Jobs, but Lower Salaries for Some. Workers are being asked to take pay cuts or face contracting-out services. In the long-term care sector in Alberta, all employees took a 5 percent pay cut to preserve their jobs. The food services personnel were then asked to take a further 12 percent cut in pay or lose their jobs to contracting-out.

The forgotten part of labour force downsizing may well be provincial ministries of health staff. The ministries' roles are changing; they are being removed from operational problems and concerns. This may result in local politicians being more aware of community concerns than the ministry.

Job Security May Be Industrywide versus Location-Specific. For union positions, regionalization in the future could bring the opportunity for job bumping throughout the region, not just within the boundaries of a facility. Bill 176, which sets out the framework for Multi-Service Agencies (MSA) in Ontario, requires that positions transferred to an MSA from a previous employer must be offered to unionized workers before non-unionized workers. This may mean non-unionized workers will take the largest hit of the re-designed long-term care service.

The Price of Receiving Union Endorsement May Be High. Unions are major stakeholders in regionalization. British Columbia conducted extensive consultation with the unions on the process of regionalization. In return for union "buy-in," a labour accord was written. The price of this accord was pay hikes in excess of other provincial comparisons, and a three-year job security arrangement. In return, the unions agreed to the disappearance of 4,000 to 5,000 jobs. The slogan became: "Save money in health care and not affect jobs."

Burnout is a Very Real Consequence in Today's Fast-Paced Reform. In 1994, Opinion Research Corp of Princeton, New Jersey surveyed middle and upper level managers about burnout:

- 68 percent of respondents saw burnout as a serious problem. More than one-third pointed to increased stress and job pressure as the main contributors. Other factors included: increased competition, higher complexity and intensity of work, the faster pace, and lay-offs and consolidations;

- almost half thought depression was on the rise among their peers;
- 64 percent were physically exhausted at the end of the day, 56 percent said that emotional exhaustion was common.

Not only are providers being asked to assume new roles, but often they must work in more than one facility. In essence they are asked to do the same job in different locations, juggle different offices and competing demands, and, be sensitive to different organizational cultures. Lay-offs affect those who stay as well as those who leave, and do contribute to burnout. Organizations need to communicate openly about changes, and work to preserve the quality of the work environment for those who remain.

Without question, Dr. Higgins and I have probably only touched the surface of the realities that are affecting health providers in this reform process. Professional autonomy, how to get input into the planning and implementation for regionalization, what is needed in persons assuming the front-line in reform, and what are the human resource consequences — these are issues and opportunities that regionalization offers.

Conclusion. Regionalization is now sufficiently entrenched in most provinces that we can turn some attention to evaluating its results. New Brunswick, first off the mark in implementing regional models is the most likely natural laboratory for a performance review of the concept. I understand that there is an openness and interest in pursuing this in New Brunswick health-care circles.

In some ways we have become obsessed with the structural issues of regionalization and have neglected the fundamental managerial questions that the health-care system still faces. For example: (i) Are costs lower? Are we actually making the system more efficient? (ii) What incentives for efficiency applied to which targets really work? (iii) Are we creating a bureaucratic organizational culture with these regions? (iv) In our efforts to be kinder and collaborative partnership oriented, are we killing off the healthy and quite fruitful effects of that good old competitive spirit? (v) Are we any further ahead on case costing funding formulae and management information system implementation in hospitals, the most expensive component of regional health systems? (vi) Are we any further ahead on comparative analysis of quality and resource utilization indicators or practice pattern variations across settings and regions?

I look forward to management and clinical leadership reasserting a managerial agenda to balance what has been almost an exclusively governance or structural agenda in regionalization initiatives to date.

CONSUMER PERSPECTIVE

Fiona Chin-Yee's Remarks

As a community activist, I have to tell you that I am angry and frustrated and that this anger fuels the passion that I feel for the communities that are looking to the stakeholder groups for leadership during these times of change. I am angry at the lack of understanding of the wisdom that people in a community bring to discussions of health care — that they are used as expendable pawns. I am angry that stakeholder groups feel that only they hold the knowledge and power to make the correct decisions and are fearful that the ignorance of the people is a major stumbling block. It is only in discussions between providers, payers, and the community that we can begin to develop a common understanding of the challenges that face us.

Regionalization is not the panacea for fixing all the problems within the health-care system — it is simply one of the tools or mechanisms to achieve a particular organizational or governance structure.

In this discussion, what is important is not "how does regionalization affect the communities?" rather, what is the "tool" of regionalization being used to do? What is the agenda, stated or unstated, that is the driving force behind regionalization?

We have been using the same words to describe radically different concepts and philosophies.

From a community perspective, we can only be included in discussions around regionalization of health services. If the driving agenda is that of decentralization of decisionmaking, it enables the appropriate decentralization of service delivery and encourages the effective use of shared services between communities and regions. Communities need to be able to take responsibility for the health of the people. Communities need to be encouraged to use the networks and resources of that community to respond to needs — only some of these resources are tied up in the health-care delivery system. Tough, ethical decisions need to be made, and it is only with the wisdom and practical experience of the people within a community that these decisions can be made and supported.

If regionalization is being used as a method to cut programs and therefore cut costs, there can be very little discussion with people in the communities because the agenda, the planning, and the direction have been set centrally; and "consulting with community groups" becomes just a meaningless activity. Regionalization, in and of itself, is not the most effective tool for cutting costs and deficit reduction. In Nova Scotia, regionalization has the effect of centralizing decisionmaking and is at risk of setting up four small central "Departments of Health" holding all decisionmaking power and inserting another layer of bureaucracy — giving very little responsibility to the communities or enabling the communities to use their own unique mix of strengths to respond to the health needs of the people.

If regionalization is being used to "de-politicize" the health-care system — the community can only be used in the most cynical of ways — deflecting attention for unpopular actions from politicians to a board of locally appointed people, this is doomed to failure. In a province with deep political roots and an understanding of both patronage and political grandstanding — a province like Nova Scotia — the people have long memories. Health care is a political reality, based on a philosophy of equal access, it is not possible or even desirable to de-politicize it. A radical shift in philosophical direction from left to right — will change our system, but this cannot be done without political ramifications.

Finally, if the regionalization of health services is structured in isolation from the governance structures of other government departments, such as Social Services, Housing, Education, Justice, then we will continue to set up reactive systems as opposed to developing proactive systems that attempt to maintain the health of the people within the community and the region.

I am no longer willing to get involved as a community activist in discussion and consultation with government departments or provider groups unless I clearly understand what the agenda driver is, what the "tool" of regionalization is attempting to achieve and how this will benefit the overall health status of the people within the community. I have to resist becoming entangled in the confusion and double-speak that has surrounded health reform and regionalization.

Stephen Learey's Remarks

When I examine the question of regionalism and decentralization, it appears that while regionalization is proceeding, we have not — as an organization — seen much evidence of decentralization. Thus, there is still centralization of decisionmaking for (i) government-appointed boards, (ii) announcements, without consultation, of hospital closures, (iii) results of commissions (which included public consultation) being shelved, and (iv) no additional funds for community services.

The community, therefore, has the perspective of an overall disappearance of services. While it is true that the matter of community boards has been addressed, we certainly feel that there should be an elective process in obtaining members. This should provide a broader representation than is currently being achieved.

We need to look at and sort through this whole process with a community perspective. Regionalization is progressing, but not decentralization. We are still seeing centralization of decisionmaking with government-appointed boards, announcements of hospital closures, and the shelving of the results of public commissions. Community services have no additional money. Services are disappearing. Community boards need to have broader representation and take part in an elective process in order to gain a wider perspective.

GENERAL DISCUSSION

Dr. Jonathan Lomas suggested three areas for discussion:

I. Opportunities for Labour Market Adjustment

There are a number of questions relating to the human resource component of the health-care system.

1. *Is regionalization taking advantage of some of the opportunities that might be offered for better labour market adjustment?*
2. *Is attention being paid to the quality of the work environment and the flexibility of the workforce?*
3. *Is labour market adjustment one of the contributors to the broader determinants of health that are the concern of the community and individuals?*
4. *Are we exploiting the potential to improve health in the community by paying attention to labour market adjustment issues?*

The payer representatives were asked to clarify the role of the regions in this activity. Here, *Dr. King* observed that regionalization could only be effective as part of an overall plan. Thus, if hospital beds were to be removed it would clearly be necessary to have some kind of community support, for example, a home-care program. Similarly, arrangements must be made to deal with the possible need to travel longer distances.

Nevertheless, it had to be recognized that there would be individuals, such as nurses, who would be displaced because of a reduction of beds. Desirably, there should be government and regional cooperation to deal with such displacement by providing appropriate training. However, it is essential to have an overall plan — not just the simple concept of regionalization.

Dr. Sullivan emphasized that money could primarily be saved by reducing the number of individuals required to accomplish specific tasks. Insufficient attention has been paid to relating training and adjustment endeavours to regional activities so that, in the most labour-intensive human services sector, a good relationship between needs and training has not yet been established.

Indeed, it appears that the only providers with employment security are physicians. Nurses and other staff who are being dislocated have no employment security despite their union status.

Dr. Higgins, being urged to comment, observed that physicians did, in fact, have to be available at all times — a sentiment that was not generally accepted. However, he noted that regionalization would introduce significant changes in the pattern of practice — both for individual physicians and in regard to referral. It had not been fully explained to potential patients that their "normal" hospital might not be available.

For physicians, it would be necessary that they acquire management skills to operate effectively in the system as a part of a team — these being fields in which they had not been trained.

Stephen Learey drew attention to the laying off of registered nurses and their replacement by lower paid, less well-trained workers. It is essential that workers should be brought into the discussion process so as to improve their overall access to employment opportunities.

At this point, discussion became general with a view expressed that labour peace could not be "bought." It had to be faced that in health care, as in many other fields, there were going to be fewer people employed — that there was not, in fact, enough useful employment to fully occupy our population.

It was also pointed out that in Nova Scotia there had not been public participation in the decisionmaking process. Hospitals were being closed without an adequate home-care program being developed. Patients were being sent home early and the system was depending on family members at home to care for elderly or invalid family members.

Dr. Lomas concluded this part of the discussion by observing that there was a feeling that human resource issues were being largely ignored. Further, there was a cascade effect in which:

- physicians were concerned that their work would be done by nurses,
- nurses saw their tasks as being given to low-paid workers or volunteers, and
- low-paid workers faced the possibility that their work would be delegated to volunteer family members.

It appeared that all these issues had not yet been incorporated into careful planning mechanisms.

II. Representation on Regional Boards

Areas of discussion:

1. *What should be the composition and representation of boards?*

2. *Should boards be elected or appointed?*

Dr. Lomas observed that there appeared to be a desire for providers to serve on regional boards, since that was where important decisions would be made. Unfortunately, their training had not dealt with this aspect of health care.

Responding, *Dr. King* noted that, when leaving medical school he had been, primarily, an "I" person. In working with a diverse range of community groups and teams it had become evident that physicians are treated differently. However, it is becoming clearer that physicians are willing to participate. He felt that with an adequate amount of training, and, given a chance to participate, physicians would be very willing to contribute.

Ms Chin-Yee felt that it was not (or had not been) an emotional matter of liking or disliking physicians, but rather that, previously, physicians did not appear to have been willing to participate in a consultation or team approach. It seemed that they demanded that their voices be heard separately — as in the various agreements made between a medical society and a province. Her view was that it was a system rather than a personal shortcoming.

Nevertheless, it was her opinion that providers should *not* sit on regional boards although they would have a very appropriate role in support groups or committees.

Stephen Learey endorsed the concept of having stakeholders involved in decisionmaking in order to get the best health results — not necessarily the best cost-cutting or government results. It is important that boards should not be a source of patronage appointments.

There was a further comment regarding the role of a board vis-à-vis management. It was beginning to appear that regional boards are perceived as all-powerful, all-knowing entities. It seemed more important to empower management so that the board, with community representation, could fulfill its appropriate role but leave the micro-management of individual facilities to managers, physicians, and clinical leaders.

At this point, *Dr. Lomas* sought to identify the three key functions for a board:

- to understand management issues and to oversee management
- to demonstrate the interests of the community with appropriate representation
- to represent important specific elements in the community, e.g., health-care providers, particular diseases or conditions, etc.

Views were sought as to the appropriate balance of these components.

Here, *Dr. King* thought it important to have all these elements represented, although recognizing that those employed by the health-care system had a conflict of interest that would prevent their serving on a board. He felt that it would be helpful to have representatives having broad views, as opposed to those representing one particular interest.

However, he suggested that provincial governments would be unlikely to turn over authority to local representatives without having their own "proxy" on the board.

Mr. Learey noted that Dr. King — a physician *and* a minister of health — demonstrated that health-care providers could serve appropriately on boards involved with decisionmaking.

III. The Role of Integration — Particularly of Primary Care

Questions for Discussion

1. *To what extent does this apply?*
2. *Is regionalization providing the funds to improve community-based primary care services?*

The intent here was to review the matter of the integration and coordination of primary care at the community level — in spite of overall central control. It does not appear, as yet, that reductions of hospital services have led to an increase in community-based services.

The community representatives noted an earlier example of a situation involving mental health where the reduction of institution activities did *not* lead to the development of a supportive environment in the community.

As well, it was pointed out that concepts could not be developed on the assumption that all regions were equal. Here there was likely to be a major issue relating to flexibility and, indeed, whether or not there would be an ability to cross provincial boundaries in order to have access to required care. Associated with this is the general question of central control, apparently of the whole range of primary care mechanisms. It is important to be clear how the health-care system would work and then to determine who, and where, the appropriate professionals would be in order to function effectively in the system.

It was asserted that primary care is a major concern to the community — it is important to take note of their needs, strengths, and required services. Thus, it seems important that providers should have a clear input to regional boards.

In a more general sense, it was considered that community health centres should be able to provide a variety of services through a range of providers (e.g., nurse practitioners) and not always through physicians. Here, it was noted that in remote or underserviced areas a physician would need such support — simply providing a cash incentive was not enough.

Dr. Lomas interceded at this point to seek guidance on what kinds of services would be appropriate for primary care, as developed by the regional authorities. Should there be something essentially different from that which exists at present?

Commenting, *Dr. King* suggested that some form of alternative payment had to be considered that would be appropriate for the individual's training and current work. He concluded that primary care physicians are advocated as the best level of access to a significant symptom or condition.

QUESTION PERIOD

At this point, the presentations and subsequent deliberations among panel members concluded and there were a number of questions from the audience.

Initially a speaker commented on the lack of reference to *patients* and posed the question of how a regionalized system would deal with a trauma victim from a motor vehicle accident. Here, it was suggested that this example was part of something greater — how to prevent the next accident, how to educate the public, etc. And, particularly, that functional regional boards with management responsibility and the support of a range of health professionals could respond better than a variety of individual efforts.

In answering the specific question it was suggested that the response would be generally the same with or without a regional board, that is, transport by ambulance to the nearest trauma centre.

The next question raised the point of how the "vision of regionalization" would contribute to the improvement of the health of Canadians. Earlier spending with vision, was bad — but replacement by "cut-backs without vision" was likely to be expensive. It would be important not to spend without a clear idea of outcomes. It was felt that it was essential to have a wide range of views on effective spending — not just the single opinions of various interest groups. Thus, the key question was how to consult with more people, to get more input and to promote a more spiritual aspect — unlike in the past where the emphasis had been on fear or self-interest.

Responding to this question *Ms Chin Yee* observed that in order to get information from the community it was important to have a community development model. The intent should not be to pose specific questions about how much to spend on this or that particular service or capital equipment, but to seek views on individuals' needs in relation to shared experiences or situations. In short, questions should be posed that would elicit the expertise or experience of individuals in the community. In this regard, questions of nutrition and understanding were more important than technical questions whose answers would be beyond them. These contentions were supported and it was noted that many elements of health care were dealt with by different government departments who were inclined not to communicate with each other. It is important to devise programs that would have a common thread and perhaps Public Health could provide the linkage in this multifaceted approach.

A member of the audience raised the question of discrimination — noting that this was now not allowed on the basis of race, religion, gender, or sexuality. It was contended, therefore, that there should be no discrimination on the basis of occupation, i.e., in particular with regard to membership on regional boards.

Dr. King noted that in New Brunswick it was accepted that physicians (not being *directly* employed by the government) could serve on boards, but not those who were employees, or part of the administrative structure. Nevertheless, the president of the medical staff could be a member but the vice-presidents medical and nursing services were only non-voting members.

Dr. Higgins supported these observations by noting that if there could be an ongoing process of interaction — as had been experienced at this roundtable — then success seemed likely. Regionalization was better than the previous system and — if not the whole answer, at least it was a beginning.

APPENDIX

Critical Issues in Regionalization

INTRODUCTION

In arranging for the topics to be dealt with at this conference it was apparent that there were many more matters that deserved consideration than there would be time available. As well, since the agenda was fairly densely packed, it was realized that there should be more opportunity for input from the range of participants.

Accordingly, it was decided to have a series of concurrent workshops that would deal with the various impacts of regionalization, i.e.,

I.   Needs-Based Planning

II.   Governance/By-Laws

IIIa. Economics/Evaluation

IIIb. Economics/Capitation Funding

IV.   Legal Accountability and Responsibility

V.   Objective Evaluation

At these workshops, individuals with the appropriate knowledge and experience outlined the key points or concerns — primarily so as to encourage a range of input and discussion from those attending. An outline of the various presentations follows.

WORKSHOP OUTLINES

I. Needs-Based Planning

Faculty: David Mowat and Bob Spasoff

Objectives:

   a. To clarify concepts and terms relevant to needs-based planning, including need, equity, efficiency, effectiveness and QALYs.

   b. To present and discuss various approaches to needs-based planning: (i) effectiveness and efficiency; (ii) public input versus evidence; (iii) desirable outcomes (as determined by the public); and (iv) how to achieve the desirable outcomes.

   c. To identify potential barriers to needs-based planning and opportunities to circumvent these barriers: (i) methodological barriers; (ii) data barriers; (iii) attitudinal barriers; (iv) political barriers.

Outline:

   a. Introduction and review of concepts.

   b. Overview of initiatives in various jurisdictions: (i) QALYs; (ii) UK NHS — Resource Allocation Working Party; (iii) Oregon; (iv) Queen's/University of Ottawa Resource Allocation Framework; (v) Ontario's District Health Councils.

   c. Practical Exercise: developing criteria to use and define required evidence; and how is information to be processed?

II. Governance/By-Laws

Faculty: John Atkinson and Lynn Curry

Objectives:

   a. To engage participants in a discussion and definition of good governance and appropriate accountability.

   b. To provide a definitional context for discussion, including a definition of governance, stakeholders, and other elements.

c. To review and discuss governance issues, including: (i) how to become a member of a regional board; (ii) the structure and function of a regional board; (iii) accountability to health-care providers, the public, the government, and the administration.

Outline:

Discussion of participants' concerns with governance issues and problems in the context of regionalization and decentralization of health care.

Discussion will then cover the following three elements:

a. How to become a board member: (i) elected or selected (advantages and disadvantages); (ii) orientation and qualifications of board members; (iii) staggered terms and criteria for adequate performance as a board member.

b. The structure and function of a regional board: (i) responsibility of the board and board members to the community and other stakeholders; (ii) hospital boards versus health boards; (iii) fiduciary responsibility; (iv) the issue of allegiances; (v) operations of the board.

c. Accountability: (i) health-care providers, the public, the government, and the administration; (ii) information and input to function (from all stakeholders); (iii) how to get organized in order to influence effectively the board.

IIIa. Economics/Evaluation

Faculty: Allan Gregory/John Dorland and Stephen Dibert/Bill Tholl

Objectives:

a. To review the basis of economic evaluation.

b. To describe the general design relating to the allocation of funds across and within regions.

c. To evaluate critically some recent regional funding approaches.

d. To design an economic evaluation protocol that allows for interjurisdictional comparisons.

Outline:

Discussion of topics:

a. Economic objectives behind regionalization, what are they and how can they be operationally defined: (i) efficiency; (ii) effectiveness; (iii) cost containment.

b. What are the strengths and limits of economic evaluation?

c. How can regionalized structures encourage better management? Are internal markets an answer?

d. The diversity of approaches to regionalization across Canada presents a unique opportunity to assess the economic impact of alternative funding approaches. What are the critical success factors to designing an economic evaluation protocol capable of accommodating this diversity?

e. Regionalization initiatives involve the significant realignment of economic incentives within the hierarchy of health decisionmaking. Who should be accountable and/or responsible for undertaking economic evaluations? (National, provincial, regional: internal or external).

IIIb. Economics/Capitation Funding

Faculty: John L. Dorland and Allan Gregory

Background: Capitation funding is a population-based system of resource allocation. Under this system resources are distributed to an entity in direct proportion to the population of that entity. The entity typically refers to a regional organizational model such as a geographically-defined local authority or a vertically-integrated corporation which serves an identified roster population. Since it is generally accepted that the need for health resources in a region is influenced by more than size, the formula also includes age and gender adjustments.

Objectives:

a. To identify the consequences of the capitation funding approach.

b. To evaluate criteria for the capitation funding approach.

c. To determine other factors for inclusion in a capitation formula.

d. To asses the strengths and weaknesses of a fee-for-service system.

Outline:

  a. Participants will meet in the Executive Decision Centre to use the state-of-the-art decision support technology along with a facilitator to focus on objectives.

  b. The "brainstorming" will use computers, but requires no computer experience.

IV. Legal Accountability and Responsibility

Faculty: Gilbert Sharpe

Objectives:

To provide participants with the opportunity to understand and explore issues of legislation and legal accountability which accompany regionalization reforms. The following issues and their legal implications will be discussed:

  a. Transfer of more responsibility for health to different types of legal structures.

  b. Interest of government in "envelope" funding on a regional/local basis.

  c. Interest in developing a list of basic services that should be provided.

  d. Widespread acknowledgement of the debt crisis and the determination by governments to reduce health-care budgets.

Outline:

  a. Discussion of the results of cutbacks in health funding such as liability of both hospitals and health professionals, and increased need for hospitals to be entrepreneurial.

  b. Discussion on use of clinical practice guidelines (CPGs) and risk-benefit ratios and their implications.

  c. Discussion regarding who makes decisions about regionalization (e.g., should they be unilateral decisions by government?). How should regional structures go about absorbing individual institutions and related issues such as medical by-laws?

V. *Objective Evaluation*

Faculty: Les Carrothers and Beverley J. Nickoloff

Objectives:

a. To provide a definitional context for objective evaluation of provincial regionalization and decentralization initiatives, based on: (i) a definition of the policy problems facing health-care planners; (ii) a definition of regionalization, decentralization, devolution, and other related terms; (iii) a review of the regionalization initiatives and instruments utilized to date in Canada.

b. To examine the application of an evaluation framework that includes questions and indicators pertaining to: (i) issues of scope, function, and transfer of authority; (ii) short-term outcomes resulting from the transfer of authority and the shift in accountability (range of available services and system management); (iii) long-term outcomes resulting from the transfer of authority and the shift in accountability (enhanced well-being of the population and cost-effectiveness).

Contributors

Malcolm Anderson is a Senior Associate in the Queen's Health Policy Research Unit at Queen's University. He is currently coordinating the Health Services Research at Queen's program. His own research includes evaluation framework development and the pharmaceutical industry.

Fiona Chin-Yee has been involved with community groups and organizations for the past 15 years and has served on many committees and task forces in Nova Scotia. Her philosophy is to advocate a system of health that looks at the broad determinants of health within a community, maximizing the potential health of community members.

Carol Clemenhagen is President of the Canadian Hospital Association. She began her career in the health-care research unit of the University of Ottawa's Department of Epidemiology and Community Medicine.

S. Mathwin Davis is an Adjunct Professor in the School of Policy Studies, Queen's University. He developed the Health Policy Specialization for the School, and is active in the governance of acute-care hospitals in Kingston and in developing an emergency plan for the city.

Raisa Deber is Professor of Health Policy in the Department of Health Administration, University of Toronto. She has written on many aspects of Canadian health policy.

John Dorland is Associate Director, Research, with the Queen's Health Policy Research Unit and is Assistant Professor in the Department of Community Health and Epidemiology. His research areas include evaluation of health-care programs, drug utilization and health information systems.

Marie Fortier has held several senior positions in Health and Welfare Canada, as well as experience as an executive director of large city hospitals. She has recently been involved in federal/provincial/territorial health activities.

Richard Fraser practises law in Alberta. His areas of specialization include health law and employment law. He is past chair of the National Health Law Section for the Canadian Bar Association and is chair of the Canadian Bar Association Task Force on Health Care Reform in Canada.

Geoffrey C. Higgins is Chief of Diagnostic Imaging at St. Clare's Mercy Hospital, St. John's Newfoundland. He has served on the CMA's Council of Health Policy and Economics and chaired the Working Group on Regionalization among other positions.

Russell H.T. King is Minister of Health and Community Services for the Government of New Brunswick. He is a member of the Cabinet Committee on Policy and Priorities. He holds the medical certification from the College of Family Physicians of Canada.

Paul LaMarche is Professor in the Department of Social and Preventive Medicine in the Faculty of Medicine at Laval University. Mr. LaMarche has experience as associate deputy minister in planning, evaluation and health in the Quebec Ministry of Health.

Léo-Paul Landry is Secretary-General of the Canadian Medical Association. His areas of concentration are: health-care policy and management and the clinical practice of medicine. He consults and teaches.

Stephen Learey is the Executive Coordinator for the Canadian Health Coalition, whose members include groups representing seniors, labour, health-care workers, anti-poverty movement and women. The Coalition has been involved in several health-care areas: The *Canada Health Act*, service cutbacks, extra-billing, user fees, and changes to the *Drug Patent Act*.

Jonathan Lomas is Professor of Health Policy Analysis in the Department of Clinical Epidemiology and Biostatistics and the coordinator of the Centre for Health Economics and Policy Analysis at McMaster

University. He is a member of the Premier's Council on Health, Well-Being and Social Justice in Ontario.

John Malcom is the CEO for the Saskatoon District Health Board. They are responsible for all aspects of health care in the district as well as health promotion, education and research.

Alan Maynard was Professor of Economics and Director of the Centre for Health Economics, York University, England. He is a member of the Economic and Social Research Council Evaluation Steering Group. His areas of study include evaluation of health service reform, primary care and addiction policy. [Since the conference took place, Alan Maynard has moved to the Nuffield Provincial Hospitals' Trust, London.]

David R. Peterson is a senior partner in the Toronto law firm of Cassels, Brock and Blackwell. He served in the Ontario Legislature from 1975 to 1990, and was premier between 1985 and 1990. He was active in Canadian constitutional discussions.

Duncan G. Sinclair is Vice-Principal (Health Sciences) and Dean of the Faculty of Medicine. He is a member of the Premier's Council on Health, Well-Being and Social Justice in Ontario and chaired the Research Steering Committee.

Terry Sullivan is President of the Institute for Work and Health, an independently incorporated, non-profit organization. He served in many senior positions in the Ontario government as well as being a member of the WHO mission to assess progress in the evolution of the Public Health Commission and health reform in New Zealand.

Alan Warren was Executive Director of the Ottawa-Carleton Regional District Health Council from its formation in 1975 until his retirement in 1995. His interests include long-term care and rehabilitation and the development of health-social service interaction.